The Essence of Play

A unique companion to professional play practice!

All play professionals are united in their belief that play is important for children's development – and there are inherent characteristics of play that underpin professional play practice across contexts. Providing an overarching concept of play, drawing together the evidence base across disciplines and linking theory to practice, *The Essence of Play* is the ideal handbook for all those working with children.

Play acts as a natural resource for children to meet physical, intellectual and emotional challenges and this book, unusually, considers play from the perspectives of children rather than adults. It provides a baseline of shared knowledge for all play professionals, exploring the fundamental value of play rather than a 'how to' approach to practice. It considers:

- the therapeutic potential inherent in play;
- how play reflects and promotes physical, emotional, intellectual, linguistic and social abilities;
- the emergence of different types of play skills and why these are important;
- cross-cultural patterns in play, gender, atypicality and adversity, highlighting the relevance of these issues to professional play practice;
- the benefits of utilising play for assessment and other professional practice issues such as ethical play practice, balancing risk with health and safety and the creation and management of boundaries.

This text is designed for students and practitioners working with children across the helping professions, including early years education, play therapy, playwork, childcare, social care, nursing and allied health. Each chapter provides directed reading and small reflective tasks to encourage readers to digest key issues.

Justine Howard is Postgraduate Programmes Manager and Senior Lecturer at the College of Human and Health Sciences at Swansea University, UK. She is a Chartered Psychologist and specialist in developmental and therapeutic play.

Karen McInnes is Senior Lecturer in the Department of Psychology at the University of Glamorgan, UK. As a trained primary school teacher and speech therapist, she previously lectured in Early Years at Bath Spa University, UK.

The Essence of Play

A practice companion for professionals working with children and young people

Justine Howard and Karen McInnes

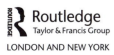

Routledge
Taylor & Francis Group

LONDON AND NEW YORK

First published 2013
by Routledge
2 Park Square, Milton Park, Abingdon, Oxon, OX14 4RN

Simultaneously published in the USA and Canada
by Routledge
711 Third Avenue, New York, NY 10017

Routledge is an imprint of the Taylor & Francis Group, an informa business

British Library Cataloguing in Publication Data
A catalogue record for this book is available from the British Library

Library of Congress Cataloging-in-Publication Data
Howard, Justine.
 The essence of play : a practice companion for professionals working
 with children and young people / Justine Howard and Karen McInnes.
  p. ; cm.
  Includes bibliographical references.
 I. McInnes, Karen. II. Title.
 [DNLM: 1. Play and Playthings—psychology. 2. Child Development.
 3. Child. 4. Play Therapy—methods. WS 105.5.P5]
 618.92′891653—dc23   2012029821

ISBN13: 978–0–415–67808–7 (hbk)
ISBN13: 978–0–415–67813–1 (pbk)
ISBN13: 978–0–203–07510–4 (ebk)

Typeset in Sabon by
Swales & Willis Ltd, Exeter, Devon

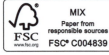

Printed and bound in Great Britain by
TJ International Ltd, Padstow, Cornwall

Contents

List of figures and tables

Figures

Tables

Foreword

I am delighted to be asked to write the Foreword for this excellent book, which I believe has the potential to really make a difference (even Narrow the Gap, to use the current mantra in the early childhood education world!). It is an optimistic book, and I hope this will be seen as an optimistic Foreword.

I was recently asked to write a report about the importance of play for the commercial organisation that represents the toy manufacturers of Europe (TIE). In that report I started by establishing the importance of play, as follows:

> Play in all its rich variety is one of the highest achievements of the human species, alongside language, culture and technology. Indeed, without play, none of these other achievements would be possible. The value of play is increasingly recognised, by researchers and within the policy arena, for adults as well as children, as the evidence mounts of its relationship with intellectual achievement and emotional well-being.
>
> Whitebread *et al.*, 2012, p. 3

As is also well documented, and reviewed in my report, children's play is under threat. The childhood I experienced, along with most of my generation, which included significant and highly memorable hours of 'playing out' with my friends in my street, and in the surrounding fields and countryside, almost entirely unsupervised by adults, has now almost completely disappeared for the vast majority of children in the UK, and in the rest of the developed world. This is a consequence, partly, of increased urbanisation, of increased perceptions of risk, and, in the educational world that I know best, of increased political involvement in education and pressure for children to achieve narrowly defined, utilitarian educational goals. Over half of the children in the world now live in cities and other urban conurbations, and many have almost no experience of the natural world. Understandably, with modern-day traffic, parents are fearful of allowing their children out to play on the streets, and also perceive a range of other risks for children in urban environments. As a consequence, these children live increasingly risk-averse lives, where they are constantly supervised and organised and their every moment is scheduled by their parents and other adults. The opportunities for free play, which I experienced almost every day of my childhood, are becoming increasingly scarce.

In the educational world other forces have also led to a deteriorating situation. When I trained to be what was then referred to as an 'Infants' teacher, in the very early 1970s, the teaching of young children was largely a quiet backwater, untroubled by any serious intellectual debate or controversy, and entirely ignored as being of no consequence by educational policy makers and politicians. British Early Years Education enjoyed an international reputation for excellence and progressive thinking, and those of us entering the profession at the time happily absorbed the well-established, and well-loved principles which had been handed down by Froebel, Montessori, Steiner, and the various other early childhood education gurus. In my own case, I was delighted to work with Dorothy Glynn (née Gardner), who had been taught herself by Susan Isaacs, and was an inspiring advocate of letting children be children, and using careful observation to provide them with whatever they needed to pursue their interests and enthusiasms (including dead birds). We were all child-centred and we unashamedly had fun!

How things have changed. When the political class finally got the message, somewhere around the late 1980s or early 1990s, that early childhood education makes a difference, all hell let loose. To begin with, this seemed a wholly positive development even if, inevitably, the arguments that persuaded them were about financial payback for the state, cutting the social services bill, efficient use of human resources, building a skilled workforce etc., rather than about the rights of children to a high-quality education and to living a happy and fulfilled life. At last, early childhood education would be taken seriously, and those of us who had been working and researching in the area of early childhood learning and pedagogy would be listened to and asked for guidance. This happened to a degree.

However, rather quickly, the situation moved in an unfortunate and counter-productive direction. If large amounts of extra taxpayers' money were going to be invested in improved early educational provision, then the accountants in the Treasury wanted to see measurable results. There had to be accountability, there had to be standards, there had to be quantifiable outcomes. Before anyone really noticed, the whole panoply of bureaucracy descended upon us, and young children had to achieve Desirable Outcomes or Early Learning Goals, all of which could be achieved by moving through ten defined stages or 'Stepping Stones' (ugh!), and all 539 of which (or was it 647?) were required to record, document, evidence and quantify by the poor, luckless saps we now must refer to as Foundation Stage practitioners. In all this, despite official protestations in some government documents to the contrary, the importance of play and having fun had been lost.

I don't think it is unreasonable to suggest that this loss of free play opportunities has, at least, in part, been a contributory factor to the alarming increase in mental health difficulties amongst children and young people in the UK in recent years. This should sound alarm bells that there are issues here which need our attention. Recent surveys, furthermore, have reported that children in the UK are the unhappiest in Europe.

While it is difficult and will take a good deal of time and investment to make our streets, towns and cities once more child-friendly, within our child-care and educational settings providing opportunities for regular, high-quality play should be relatively straightforward. However, despite some of the rhetoric, the argument in this area still needs to be won. In this arena, in my view, a large part of the problem has been that those of us involved in early childhood education have been ill-equipped to defend our belief in the importance of play. We all know that children respond best when they were in a loving and warm environment, that they are more involved in tasks when they had chosen them freely for themselves, and that they learn best through play, but we have not been really sure why any of this is the case or how this all works. The kind of hard, quantifiable and rigorous research that is understood by accountants and politicians had not been done, because there was never been a need. And where it had been done, it was not widely disseminated and understood by many in the early childhood workforce. So, often, when the politicians have asked for the evidence that children would not learn better by being required to learn by rote, it has not been forthcoming.

While the importance of play for children's learning and well-being has been widely recognised for many years, developing practices within early years settings which support children's play in the most beneficial ways has often proven to be very difficult. A number of projects have documented the lack of productive play opportunities in early years classrooms and settings, despite the avowed enthusiasm for learning through play expressed by the practitioners involved. The policy documentation in this area has also been redolent with misconceived notions, such as 'planned, productive play', which has spectacularly missed the key point that play, in its very essence, is unplanned and spontaneous. This lack of effective play practice in educational settings has been damaging for the education of the children involved, of course, but has also been damaging in dividing the community of adults who work with young children. The failure of many adults working with children to play with them effectively has been misconstrued as evidence that play must be adult free, rather than that adults need to be able to play. This has led to an unfortunate polarisation of views between those in the recreational and therapeutic play communities, who regard adult involvement in children's play as anathema, or certainly the adult direction of play as unhealthy, and those in the educational world who see children's natural playfulness as an opportunity for adults to provide stimulating and effective learning opportunities.

By turning conventional thinking on its head, and seeing play from the perspective of the children, rather than that of the adults, however, Howard and McInnes show, in this wonderful book, how recent research evidence can provide new insights into the fundamentals of play practice within educational, recreational and therapeutic settings. Central to this is their own innovative research and insights into the play cues that children use in order to decide if an activity is playful or not, combined with the crucial evidence that activities perceived as playful evoke improved involvement, perseverance and performance, compared to identical activities which are presented in a way which makes them appear not playful. This is a stunning insight. Equally important, however, is the revelation that, in some settings, the involvement or presence of an adult leads children to perceive the activity as not playful, while in other settings this is not a relevant consideration. This speaks volumes about the practice in these different settings. And then, brilliantly, Howard and McInnes go on to analyse the practice in those settings where adults can play effectively with children, and the enhanced playful opportunities that this affords. Much of the book then documents clear guidelines, based on this seminal research, to high-quality playful practice which is relevant in any play setting, be it of a recreational, therapeutic or educational nature. In doing so, the authors have performed a vitally important service to the play community, and particularly to the young children with which we all work. This book deserves to have enormous influence, and I very much hope it does. I do believe that Howard and McInnes have, in this important field, discovered the play world's equivalent of the Higgs boson (finally discovered today!): it gives everything else weight. It took 50 years to find the elusive particle which glues together everything in the Universe, and for Professor Higgs to be put forward for a Nobel prize. We can only hope that the present authors' contribution is recognised more quickly!

David Whitebread
Cambridge
July 2012

Acknowledgements

We are grateful to everyone who has supported us in writing this book. Our writing is brought to life by the stories and experiences shared with us by friends, students, colleagues and practitioners. Most photographs that appear in the book belong to the authors, and we are very grateful to have received permission to use these pictures from all who are featured. The hospital play photographs were provided by Lisa Morgan, and we extend a special thanks to her for these.

Introduction

We have both spent considerable time working as practitioners in children's services before moving into academic research and teaching positions within higher education, specialising in play and child development and their relationship to practice.

Throughout our time as practitioners we were and remain passionate about the role of play for children's health and happiness, and we have sought to forefront this in our work. We have both utilised play as a means of developing relationships with the children with whom we have worked, as an ongoing form of communication and as a way to maximise children's developmental potential.

We are fortunate that we are now in a position to share our enthusiasm about children's play through the undergraduate, postgraduate and continuing professional development courses that we teach. However, we have both been frustrated that the important academic disciplines, and professional fields within children's services seem not to share information with each other in terms of seeking parallels in their findings or reflections on play practice. In particular, there seems debate about a focus on the 'here and now' benefits of play and its 'developmental function'. We certainly do not negate the here-and-now benefits of play. We both understand the value of this. Indeed, as you will see when you read through the book, our thoughts are that the 'here and now' benefits of play are inextricably linked to its role in maximising 'developmental potential' across domains.

We believe that sharing information about what might help to ensure children's health and wellbeing is not something we have a right to be precious about. We are all working towards the same goal. While there may be differences in the training opportunities we have each pursued, our end goal is always the same – for children to be and become whatever it is that they wish, and to be happy and healthy as they pursue this life-long journey.

Children learn in lots of different ways – by imitation and modelling; through praise and reinforcement; by memorising and rote – but there is something special about their learning through play. In this book, we hope to synthesise research findings from a number of academic disciplines as well as from various studies that reflect on professional practice. Our aim is to use this information to provide all professionals within children's services with a strong, unified foundation as to what it is about play that makes it unique and extraordinarily valuable for children's development.

The message in our book appears a very simplistic one. It doesn't so much matter what an activity looks like, it's what it feels like to the child that is all-important. Play is where children feel they are in control, where they are doing what they want, following their own line of thinking and trying out their own actions and ideas. It is about being, and feeling, playful. However, facilitating this challenges us as professionals on a number of levels. Firstly, we need to know what play is and what makes it different from other activities children might engage in. What makes an activity play or not play from a child's point of view, how can we find this out and what difference does this make to how they behave? We need to step away from any outcomes we might associate with the activities we have planned for the children in our care. Outcomes must be secondary to our understanding that a sense of playfulness is all-important. Finally, and perhaps most problematic, is that we need to accept that if the benefits of play are associated with children' s own self-initiated and self-directed activity, the developmental and therapeutic potential of an activity can occur in any context and at any time. This is something that as children's service professionals we must all be attuned to.

Contemporary research convincingly demonstrates that the characteristics of play that make it so valuable for children's development are that it affords autonomy and control, thus promoting emotional regulation, confidence and self-esteem. This in turn influences all other areas of development. The emotional contribution of play to children's development is crucial and no longer a topic confined to the therapy room. The principles of playwork practice and the principles of non-directive play therapy are based on choice and control, and research findings evidencing effective practice in health care and educational settings resonate with this. All play professionals are united in their belief that play is important to children's development and that the developmental and therapeutic potential inherent in play does not distinguish between the contexts in which children engage.

Policy documentation in the UK and beyond emphasises a multi-disciplinary approach to children's services. It is time for us to reconsider our roles, to reconcile the knowledge base that underpins our work, the work of others and all of our experiences of play practice. The time has come to truly reflect on what all practitioners must understand about play in order for us to provide the best-quality experiences for the children in our care. The best quality of care depends on a thorough understanding of the research evidence relating to play and a personal philosophy as to why play is important.

Rather than proposing that play does something unique or something irreplaceable, we offer a pragmatic (but nonetheless a very powerful) view. We propose that play is like a loudspeaker, an amplifier, maximising all of the learning processes that we know already are at work. Quite simply, children learn and develop more effectively when they learn and develop through play; when they are being and feeling playful.

A feature of our book is that we focus on what separates play from others types of activity, namely playfulness. We propose that the autonomy and control children are afforded in activities they define as play creates a fear-free environment that allows them to try out new ideas, test boundaries and take risks in their own self-regulated space. Essentially these characteristics are at the heart of play practice in health, education, recreation and therapeutic contexts. Play acts as a resource for children to meet and overcome intellectual and emotional challenge.

Building on the work of Bronfenbrenner (1979), Hendry and Kloep (2002) argue that development occurs as a result of interaction between the challenges we face and the resources we have available to meet these challenges. Based on this framework, Howard (2010c) argues that play serves as one of many resources pools that influence children's ability to meet intellectual and emotional challenge. The characteristics inherent in play, which separate it from other modes of action, namely the child's perception of autonomy, control and independence, create a low-risk environment for the development of skills and dispositions that contribute to intellectual and emotional intelligence. We demonstrate the benefits of adopting a playful approach throughout the book in relation to problem-solving, self-regulation and emotional wellbeing.

The challenge-resource model of play (as depicted in Figure 0.1) proposes a relationship between the level of play resources available to the child and the complexity of the challenge being faced, which in turn determines the level of anxiety experienced and amount of support they might require (Howard, 2010c).

All children need to play, but not all children need play therapy: most can deal with the challenges they face in life through their own spontaneous play and a nurturing environment (McMahon, 2009). However, for some children, the volume or intensity of adverse situations can be overwhelming, and additional well-considered support is required. This might include play therapy, occupational therapy, play in a hospital environment, the provision of additional or focused play opportunities in a social care or school context, recreational play activities or parent–child play sessions in the community. These practices can involve working in small groups where children can benefit from peer support and shared experience or on a one-to-one basis. Protective factors such as secure attachment bonds, empathic and consistent care and appropriate play experiences increase children's resilience, and play can function on a remedial and preventative level. Masten and Coatsworth (1998) propose that vulnerability to risk can be reduced by (1) removing the risk or working to reduce its subsequent impact via preventative techniques or (2) adding resources, such as additional play provision, to reduce or counterbalance impact.

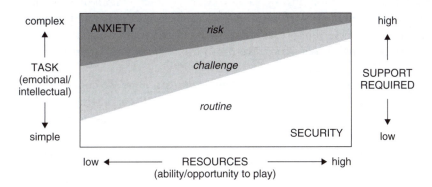

Figure 0.1 Challenge-resource model of play

We aim to identify how children's play develops and how they develop as they play. The way that play reflects and promotes children's physical, emotional, intellectual, linguistic and social ability is considered. We look at the emergence of different play skills and why each of these developmental play skills is important. We look at diversity and difference in play, with a particular emphasis on professional play practice issues. Play as an effective means of naturalistic assessment and documentation is considered, as is the creation and management of the play space, play materials and professional play practice issues such as safeguarding and risk. Within the book we pose questions that are aimed at developing practitioners' thinking about play as well as their practice, and suggestions for further reading are provided.

A brief overview of each chapter now follows:

Chapter 1 looks at theoretical perspectives of play. We begin by identifying and discussing some of the early philosophical theories of play and then draw on theorists from each of the recognised play practices: educational, recreational and therapeutic. We provide an overview of each theorist in relation to their key ideas regarding play, their definition of play and how this relates to the child. We end by looking at theorists who cross play–practice boundaries and advocate a view of play that can be shared by all play practitioners.

Chapter 2 looks at development and play. We identify theories of learning and how these relate to theories of play. We look at child development and how play enhances development from birth to adolescence, and we consider the development of play and how this might be promoted.

Chapter 3 is where we really introduce the idea of playfulness as distinct from play. We anticipate that practitioners may find this chapter difficult as it turns on its head recognised thinking about play. It also relies on practitioners viewing children as active agents in their lives with voices that need to be heard. It is this view that underpins the concept of playfulness provided here – that we need to understand play from children's perspectives, not our own. It is only once we do that that we can provide children with experiences that allow them to be playful and benefit from engaging in playful activities. This chapter is underpinned by recent and ongoing research into children's perspectives of play.

In Chapter 4 we look at the role of the adult in promoting play. We identify how children's perceptions of the adult during play are critical to their overall perception of play, and how the adult interacts with children during play may or may not facilitate playfulness. We discuss a cycle of play that is dependent upon accurate and appropriate reading of, and responding to, play cues. We finish the chapter with discussion of a process for reflecting on play practice.

Chapter 5 provides a discussion on the play environment. Here we consider some features of the play environment such as the type of places and spaces where children like to play and some of the important developmental benefits associated with particular play types and materials.

Chapter 6 is concerned with diversity and play. We provide and understanding of inclusion and how inclusion and diversity relates to play policy and provision. We look at different aspects of diversity in relation to play, for example, gender, culture and disability. We then discuss the value of play in overcoming diversity.

Chapter 7 begins with a discussion of how play provides an important medium for observation and assessment and why practitioners need to engage with this. We introduce basic observation strategies and useful measures for assessing different elements of play. By using case studies, we sensitively highlight how easy it is to misread children's play cues, and demonstrate the importance of careful observation and assessment to really understand children at play.

In Chapter 8 we look at professional practice issues common to all play practitioners, including health and safety, ethical issues and working with parents. We draw on good practice from across various professional contexts so that we can learn from one another and identify common elements of our work.

In the conclusion of our book we outline seven evidenced benefits of play, which we hope will give you confidence in your professional practice. We reiterate our position that emotional wellbeing provides the foundation for learning and development across domains and that play is a key way to support this.

We are convinced that all play practitioners need to learn from one another and find common ground to provide the best play experiences for children, which will benefit them not only in the here and now, but also in the future. We believe the starting point for this is to have a shared theoretical understanding of play based on playfulness, which can only be gained from listening to what children say about play. Basing the play experiences we provide on an adult understanding of play, we are likely to remain frustrated by the limitations of our efforts. We are convinced that the way forward for all professionals who engage in play with children is to talk with one another and learn from our experiences. We hope that this book will provide the beginning of that dialogue and maximise the opportunities to be playful for both practitioners and, most importantly, children.

1 Theoretical perspectives on play

Aims of the chapter

- To discuss different types of play practice.
- To identify the theories and theorists underpinning the different play practices.
- To discuss how this results in a lack of shared practice among play practitioners.
- To identify points of common practice between play practitioners.

Introduction

Play has been the subject of theoretical musings throughout history. Since the time of Aristotle and Plato, the value and benefits of play have been debated and discussed, and different viewpoints and definitions have been put forward (Cohen, 2006). Consequently, there is not one, clear theoretical view or definition of play. This chapter will acknowledge this theoretical diversity by identifying theorists of play and their unique contribution to our growing understanding of play. However, instead of taking a chronological approach to developing play theory this chapter will look at how theory has developed and underpinned different play practices. It will identify the theorists who have contributed to the theory underpinning educational, therapeutic and recreational play practice. It will look at how these theorists have defined play and their key ideas about play, and where there is overlap between ideas and different play practices. It will also consider how these different theoretical standpoints have contributed to our view of children and how we engage in play practice with them. It will also identify those rare theorists who cannot be pigeonholed as their ideas cross all play practice boundaries.

There are many theories and theorists of play, each one emphasising a slightly different view of play and the value and benefits that might be derived from engaging in play activities. All types of play practice are based on theoretical understanding. There are considered to be three distinct play practices: educational, therapeutic and recreational (Sheridan, Howard & Alderson, 2011), and practitioners within each of these categories tend to understand and value play in different ways. Educational play practitioners tend to value play as tool to aid learning and development (e.g. F. P. Hughes, 2010). Therapeutic play practitioners tend to value play as a medium of communication to enable social and emotional growth in children facing difficult life events (Axline, 1979), while recreational play practitioners value the inherent freedom that children have as they engage in play (Else, 2009). Each of these types of play practitioner draw on relevant and appropriate theory to support their view of play. At times the theorists and theories utilised are unique to that type of play practice, for example, Klein [1882–1960] and therapeutic play practice while others cross practice boundaries, for example, Sutton-Smith (1997). These theorists of play also tend to have slightly different definitions of play.

Defining play is fraught with difficulty. It means different things to different people (Howard, 2002), with some commentators of play stating that play is impossible to define (Moyles, 1989), although many of the theorists discussed below have made the attempt. Theorists such as Piaget (1951) defined play according to categories of practice play, symbolic play and games with rules, while Hughes (2006) has identified different play types. Others have tried to define play according to criteria or dispositions such as play being pleasurable and voluntary (e.g. Rubin, Fein & Vandenberg, 1983). However, these ways of defining play are not necessarily helpful to play practitioners. Most play practitioners discuss creating the right conditions or context for children's play (e.g. Brown, 2008), while others identify play as a behaviour or types of behaviours (e.g. Burghardt, 2011). Many play practitioners view play as a disposition or a way of being emphasising the positive sense of self and wellbeing that comes with play (e.g. Isaacs, 1929). This is often viewed alongside a definition of playfulness, something that is viewed as separate from play (e.g. Dewey, 1933). All play practitioners would probably agree that play is a process, and many theorists discuss play in this way. But this opens up as many definitional problems as it solves. How the process is defined and what exactly constitutes the process probably mean different things to different people. In discussing theorists of play their definitions will be considered according to whether they view play as behaviour, context or disposition as well as process, and how this influences play practice.

Historically, children have been perceived in different ways dependent upon the prevailing views and needs of the time – from Locke's view of the child as a *tabula rasa* to Rousseau's view of childhood as an age of innocence. In more recent times children and childhood have been viewed as a social and cultural construction, with debate concerning whether children are viewed as a progressing through a natural state on the way to adulthood (becomings) or as individuals in their own right (beings) (James, Jenks & Prout, 1998). There are some who view children as both beings in the here and now and as becomings given the natural development and growth that children go through (Lee, 2002). According to current discourses, children are seen as active agents in their lives, should have a say in their lives and be heard by those who work with them (James *et al.*, 1998). In addition, Dahlberg, Moss and Pence (2007) state that views of childhood and children are 'productive of practice' (p. 52), and this can be seen in the way that play theorists influence practice and ultimately the view of the child. The discussion of theorists below will identify the likely view of the child, as being or becoming, implied from their theoretical position on play.

Theorists and theories of play

The following discussion of theorists and theories of play will be primarily organised according to type of play practice: educational, therapeutic and recreational. Some theorists cannot be categorised in this way, and they will be identified and discussed separately. There are also those classical, philosophical theories that are cited by all, irrespective of play practice. These theories provide a starting point for any theoretical discussion of play despite having limited application to the theorists and theories that have followed, but in terms of historical referencing they are important.

Classical theories of play

These early philosophical theories of play have previously been presented as opposing pairs (Saracho & Spodek, 1998). The surplus energy theory of play proposed by Spencer [1820–1903] stated that play was a product of superfluous energy left over after all other basic needs had been met. While the relaxation theory of play by Lazarus [1824–1903] took an opposing view, rather than seen as using surplus energy, play was an activity that occurred after work in order to relax and build up further energy. The recapitulation theory of play by Hall [1846–1924] saw the function of play as cathartic in that through playing children acted out evolutionary stages, while the pre-exercise theory by Groos [1861–1946] explained play as an opportunity to practise adult activities and prepare for adult life. Certainly these types of activities can be seen in children's play today, and many early years education practitioners will justify play in the curriculum in this way.

All of these theories may be considered as a reflection of the time period in which they were proposed. They are all defining play as a behaviour or an activity in which children naturally engage. As a naturally occurring behaviour there would be little consideration of the context of play or play as a disposition. The view of the child implied by these different theories is also a reflection of the times. The first two theories

Table 1.1 Classical theories of play

Theorist	Key ideas	Definition of play	View of child
Spencer 1820–1903	Product of excess energy	Behaviour	Being
Lazarus 1824–1903	A form of relaxation after work	Behaviour	Being
Hall 1846–1924	Cathartic, play out evolutionary stages	Behaviour	Being and Becoming
Groos 1861–1946	Preparation for adult life	Behaviour	Being and Becoming

imply that childhood is a time of being, with no sense of becoming. In the early 1800s children were expected to help with the daily life of the family from a young age. They were often exploited to the detriment of their education. However, by the late 1800s young children's education was taken more seriously, and there was a recognition that education would provide a more effective workforce later on (Fawcett, 2000). Hence, the two later theories may be considered as viewing children not just as beings but also as becomings through the cathartic and skill-based experience of play. An overview of these theories is provided in Table 1.1.

Theorists of educational play practice

Froebel [1782–1853] is a key theorist underpinning early years education. He invented the first kindergarten (literally, young children's garden) in Germany and saw play as central to children's learning and development. He espoused open-ended, real experiences for children without rules imposed on them by others – quite different to views of play within education today and more in keeping with recreational play practice. Froebel saw play as an integrating mechanism that brought all aspects of development together. He developed his Occupations – a range of craft-like activities and Gifts – a set of wooden blocks with endless possibilities for open-ended play and learning (Bruce, 2011). Froebel's view of play may be defined as a disposition, behaviour and process as children are able to wallow in play as well as developing through play, hence both being and becoming.

Dewey [1859–1952] is often mentioned in educational texts but rarely in texts on play. However, he was possibly the first theorist to clearly differentiate playfulness from play. He stated that 'the former is an attitude of mind; the latter is an outward manifestation of this attitude' (Dewey, 1933, p. 210). In this way it would seem that he saw play as a behaviour and playfulness as a disposition. This view would have resonance with both therapeutic play practice, where theorists also emphasise playfulness in a similar way, and with recreational play practice through play as behaviour. As an educationalist he saw education, and presumably play, as a means for growth, so viewing childhood as a time of becoming.

Like Froebel, Montessori [1870–1952] is a key theorist underpinning early years education. However, her views on play are less in keeping with current early years play practice. She saw play and work as synonymous, usually referring to work as the child's life in progress, which the teacher should respect and enhance (Montessori, 1965); this would lead to growth of the child, hence she saw the child as becoming. She believed that children should have freedom to choose what to play, but children were taught to use materials in a didactic way and not use them in any other way, a far cry from recognised play practice. By using carefully graded materials in a set way children were then free to learn by themselves.

Susan Isaacs [1885–1948] was a psychologist who was also influential within the development of early years education. She valued the practical activities and interactions children engaged in while playing as these supported a positive sense of self, which would lead to intellectual development. However, Isaacs also valued children's spontaneous play, especially play without adults, as children may behave differently and by observing adults could gain new insights into the child (Isaacs, 1932). In this way her view of children could be interpreted as being and becoming. The emphasis on the positive sense of self through play is shared with therapeutic play practice.

Piaget [1896–1980] was also a psychologist whose ideas have been influential within education. His theory of play (1951) was an extension of his work on intellectual development. He also defined a stage theory of play that reflected levels of intellectual development. Piaget's concept of play derived from his concept of assimilation, and he saw play as secondary to learning such that through play children could secure what they already knew.

Writing at the same time as Piaget was another psychologist, Vygotsky [1896–1934]. He took a different view from Piaget in placing greater emphasis on the social and cultural aspects of play. He saw play as a form of language and communication, arguing that play promoted cognitive, emotional and social development (Bodrova & Leong,

Table 1.2 Theorists informing educational play practice

Theorist	Key ideas	Definition	View of child	Links to other play practice
Froebel 1782–1852	Open-ended play, play as an integrating mechanism	Behaviour, disposition and process	Being and Becoming	Recreational play
Dewey 1859–1952	Play and playfulness	Behaviour and disposition	Becoming	Therapeutic play and recreational play
Montessori 1870–1952	Learn by themselves, freedom to choose	Work synonymous with play	Becoming	
Isaacs 1885–1948	Positive sense of self, intellectual development	Behaviour, disposition and context	Being and Becoming	Therapeutic play
Piaget 1896–1980	Stage theory of play, secondary to learning	Behaviour	Becoming	
Vygotsky 1896–1934	Imaginative play, form of language and communication	Behaviour and process	Becoming	Therapeutic play
Bruner 1915–	Modes of exploration for learning	Behaviour and context	Becoming	Recreational play

2007). Vygostsky is often quoted as saying that play is the leading activity for young children, but what is often missed is that Vygostsky valued imaginative play and that his criterion for defining play was that it must have an imaginary situation (Vygotsky, 1933). From the emphasis on development it would seem that his view of children would be as becoming, and his emphasis on play as a form of communication would be shared with theorists of therapeutic play practice.

The views of both Piaget and Vygotsky have been synthesised in the work of Bruner [1915–]. He devised three forms of exploration: enactive, iconic and symbolic, which children use to explore the world and develop; therefore he viewed children as becoming. He saw that play provided a safe environment and conditions in which children could explore, hence play as context, but he also thought that play enabled children to try out new combinations of behaviour (Bruner, 1972), a view shared with theorists of recreational play. For a synopsis of theorists of educational play practice, see Table 1.2.

Theorists of therapeutic play practice

Therapeutic play practice derives from the psychoanalytic tradition of Sigmund Freud [1856–1939]. He thought there was a strong relationship between imaginative play and creativity, and that through the context of play children would play out traumatic events, thereby gaining mastery over them. He believed that through play children developed emotionally; therefore his view of children would be as becoming. Anna Freud [1895–1982] developed her father's work. As well as play enabling children to overcome traumatic events she also believed that the context of play provided a means to establish a relationship between the therapist and child, and that this would facilitate the process of psychotherapy. She also thought that through children playing in therapy they would talk about conscious feelings and thoughts and act out unconscious conflicts (McMahon, 2009).

Building on Anna Freud's work, Klein [1882–1960] saw children's play as the equivalent of free association. She saw play as indicative of conflict, which they communicated from their unconscious mind. The job of the therapist was to interpret their play behaviour and ease conflict. In addition, Klein was probably the first therapist to use a carefully planned play room in which the child was free to choose and direct their own play (McMahon, 2009).

Winnicott [1896–1971] shared Freud's view that there was a link between play and creativity. Like Vygotsky, he saw play as a form of communication, firstly between the mother and child and then between the therapist and child. He believed that communication occurred in the playful space between these two people (Winnicott, 1971). The idea of a playful space has links with recreational play practice. Winnicott disagreed with Klein's view that play needed to be interpreted, and thought rather that children needed to be allowed to play, be creative and discover themselves.

Erikson [1902–1994] studied with Anna Freud and saw play as healing. Like Isaacs, he thought that through play children developed a positive sense of self, a sense of competence and self-esteem, which occurred through the first three years. However, unlike Isaacs, he did not link this to intellectual development.

Axline [1911–1988] is an inspirational figure for most therapeutic play practitioners who first learn about play therapy through her book *Dibs: In Search of Self* (Axline,

1979). Building on the work of Rogers (1951), she believed that children had the power to solve their own problems through play in the right therapeutic environment. Axline developed non-directive play therapy whereby children were free to play within the contained space of the play room. Through playing the child communicated his or her thoughts and feelings, and the therapist's role was to reflect these back to the child so they could gain insight into themselves (McMahon, 2009). The idea of play being free from adult direction has resonance with recreational play practice.

Sue Jennings is a play and drama therapist who utilises a therapeutic practice based on creativity. She developed the Embodiment-Projection-Role (EPR) developmental play model, which charts the development of dramatic play from birth to 7 years of age. The notion of development through dramatic play has shared links with current educational play practice. For an overview of theorists of therapeutic play practice, see Table 1.3.

Table 1.3 Theorists informing therapeutic play practice

Theorist	Key ideas	Definition of play	View of child	Links to other play practice
Freud, S. 1856–1939	Imaginative play, play through traumatic events	Context and behaviour	Becoming	
Freud, A. 1895–1982	Enables a relationship between therapist and child, explore emotions	Context and process	Becoming	
Klein 1882–1960	Play indicative of conflict, needs interpreting	Context and process	Becoming	
Winnicott 1896–1971	Creation of a playful space between therapist and child	Context and process	Being and Becoming	Recreational play
Erikson 1902–1994	Play develops a sense of competence and self-esteem	Context and disposition	Becoming	
Axline 1911–1988	Non-directive play, under the child's direction and choice	Context and process	Being and Becoming	Recreational play
Jennings	Developmental play and the EPR model	Behaviour and context	Being and Becoming	Educational play

Theorists of recreational play

Desmond Morris [1928–] has discussed play as a behaviour and argued that humans possessed an innate drive to play (Else, 2009). This enabled humans to discover and get to know the world. In this way Morris was discussing play in the here and now, and hence has a view of children as beings.

Burghardt [1941–] has taken an all-encompassing view of play, looking at play in both animals and humans. He states that play needs to be defined, and his definition can be utilised for both animals and humans. He has developed five criteria that, taken together, enable an observer to recognise play behaviour. The criteria cover both play as a behaviour and as a disposition (Burghardt, 2011). He has also developed a hierarchy of play that outlines play as a developmental process (Burghardt, 2005); this has links with educational play practice, and as such children may be viewed as both beings and becomings.

Hughes [1944–] is a playworker who has defined playwork as the essence of wild play experience free from adult interference, which is then brought into an artificial setting, for example, an adventure playground (B. Hughes, 2011). He emphasises the importance of the play environment for play behaviour to occur.

Sturrock [1948–] views play from a variety of academic disciplines: psychology, education, playwork and play therapy. Drawing on this varied background he has outlined the importance of playwork for enabling children to work out potential neuroses (Else, 2009) and has combined recreational and therapeutic play practice to create 'psycholudics', which is the study of the mind and psyche at play (Ludemos Associates, 2008–11). Based on this work Sturrock has created a new terminology, which is used by recreational play professionals. For an overview of theorists of recreational play practice, see Table 1.4.

Table 1.4 Theorists informing recreational play practice

Theorist	Key ideas	Definition of play	View of child	Links to other play practice
Morris 1928–	Play behaviour is an innate drive, get to know the world	Behaviour	Being	
Burghardt 1941–	Playfulness in animals and humans, hierarchy of play	Behaviour, disposition and process	Being and Becoming	Educational play
Hughes 1944–	Importance of adult free play	Behaviour, context and process	Being	
Sturrock 1948–	Own terminology – psycholudics, children 'play out' neuroses	Behaviour, context and process	Being and Becoming	Therapeutic play

Theorists crossing boundaries

There are two key theorists of play whose theories cross play practice boundaries. Sutton-Smith [1924–] is a psychologist who writes about play from a variety of perspectives for an audience interested in play. He has derived seven rhetorics of play, which encompass both children's and adult's play. These and reflect different functions of play such as play as progress, a developmental perspective and play of the self whereby play is viewed as escapism, for fun and relaxation (Sutton-Smith, 1997). His all-encompassing writing about play as enabling flexibility and variability means play may be viewed as context, behaviour, disposition and process. Sutton-Smith advocates children making their own decisions during play as well as giving consideration to their view of what constitutes play. It is possible to discern in his writing a view of children as both being and becoming.

Garvey is also a psychologist whose writing is for a varied audience interested in play. She was keen to define play, and created five characteristics of play that encompass play as a disposition, a process and behaviour (Garvey, 1991). She also emphasised the social and communicative context of play. She highlighted the developmental function of play, although she believed that play promoted all aspects of development. Garvey also advocated that children should be allowed to play free from adult interference, whereby the adult role was to observe and learn. In this way her writing crosses the boundaries of educational, therapeutic and recreational play practice, and her view of children is of them both being and becoming. Table 1.5 gives a synopsis of these two play theorists.

Conclusion

This chapter has identified different theoretical positions concerning play and childhood underpinning the different play practices. It has identified those rare theorists who

Table 1.5 Theorists crossing boundaries

Theorist	Key ideas	Definition of play	View of child	Links to other play practice
Sutton-Smith 1924–	Ambiguities of play for children and adults, different functions of play, children making their own decisions	Behaviour, context, disposition and process	Being and Becoming	Educational, therapeutic and recreational play practice
Garvey	Characteristics of play, social engagement, all areas of development	Behaviour, context, disposition and process	Being and Becoming	Educational, therapeutic and recreational play practice

cross practice boundaries, and has demonstrated the value for all play practitioners in crossing theoretical and, therefore, practice boundaries. By doing this all play practitioners can value and learn from each other and facilitate play opportunities that benefit all children across developmental domains.

Our own theoretical position concerning play will be demonstrated in the following chapters. We will discuss our belief that playfulness, rather than the play act itself, is the key ingredient that benefits children. Our discussion on playfulness will highlight the importance of children feeling like an activity is play regardless of how adults might perceive that activity. Building on the ideas of flexibility and fluency proposed by Bruner and Sutton-Smith, feeling playful means that children feel able to try out new ideas and resolve conflicts and anxieties in a safe way. These ideas will be discussed in subsequent chapters by utilising more recent ideas such as compound flexibility (Brown, 2003) and a threshold and fluency model of play (Howard, 2010a).

Now that you have read the chapter

- How do you view play? Write your own definition of play using 20 words or less.
- Analysing your definition of play, what does it tell you about how you view play?
- Which theories of play contribute to your understanding of play and your view of children? After reading the chapter, do you need to reconsider how you view play?
- If you work in a team, facilitate a team discussion on play and children. Do all members of the team understand play and children in the same way? Do you need to spend some time developing a shared understanding of play and children that may form the basis for a play policy that may be shared with other practitioners and parents?

Useful further reading

Cohen, D. (2006) *The Development of Play*, 3rd edn (London: Routledge), Chapter 2: A history of play (pp. 14–32).
This chapter provides a clear narrative of the historical underpinnings of play, mainly from an educational and psychological perspective. It also identifies how various theorists saw the value of play for different domains of development.

Else, P. (2009) *The Value of Play* (London: Continuum), Chapter 9: A play history – From Plato to the play ethic (pp. 140–153).
A useful and readable chapter, which provides a chronological overview of different theorists and their contribution to play practice.

2 Exploring play and child development

Aims of the chapter

- To explore some of the theories that help us to understand the ways in which children develop and learn.
- To outline particular milestones in children's development from birth through to adolescence, including the development of their play.
- To explore the ways in which play offers opportunities for children to develop and learn.
- To highlight the value of play as a means of enhancing children's development across domains, introducing the concept of playfulness as a means of achieving this.

Introduction

The systematic study of how children think and learn is relatively new. French historian Ariès (1960, p. 4) wrote that in the Middle Ages to pre-modern times children were treated very much like miniature adults, and childhood was not really considered as a developmental period worthy of scientific attention. Children wore adult clothes, worked from an early age and participated in adult-like pastimes. Little was really known about child development and there was much speculation. For example, the notion that a child was fully formed inside of the male sperm prior to implantation, with development comprising merely growth in size and bulk, was not contested until advances in microscopy enabled scientists to examine sequential foetal growth (Crain, 2005). This 'pre-formationist' view was even depicted in the artwork of Leonardo da Vinci (see his sketches of the foetus *in utero*). As well as increased scientific knowledge and understanding, a number of other factors fed our interest in the systematic study of children. These included religious drives toward education, industrialisation and the growing impact of market forces.

At the start of what has been termed the 'Age of Enlightenment', two philosophers had a particularly profound impact on views of children and childhood and, arguably, the contrasting ideas they proffered not only influenced the scientific study of child development throughout the twentieth century, but are also echoed in theoretical positions to this day. Locke [1632–1704] proposed that children were born *tabula rasa*, or blank slates, upon which perceptual experiences could be imprinted, the environment moulding the mind and learning being based on association, repetition, imitation, reward and punishment. In contrast, Rousseau [1712–1778] saw the child as a 'noble savage', having a behavioural repertoire that was inclined to act on impulse and drive toward natural curiosity. This impulsivity could be shaped and harnessed via social forces, but this shaping was reliant on elements of developmental growth at particular stages of childhood such as: sensory learning in infancy; the growth of independence and emergent reasoning in early childhood; physical growth and cognitive development of middle childhood; and finally the emergence of the social being in adolescence.

The ideas of Locke and Rousseau sparked enthusiasm for understanding children's development. Charles Darwin and Wilhelm Preyer became known as baby biographers, documenting the development of their own children in great detail. Their work was highly influential in the laboratory studies of child development conducted by James Baldwin, and all of these influenced the well-known work of Piaget. We began to consider the impact of early experiences on children's development, something reflected in the contentious ideas of Freud. In essence, early philosophical ideas:

- changed thinking about childhood and elevated it as a separate and unique period in the lifespan;
- initiated debate as to whether development was a result of nature or nurture;
- asked us to consider whether some elements of child development are stage-like (echoed in the work of Freud, Erikson, Bruner and Piaget);
- raised the idea that early experiences may be important (as can be seen in the work of Freud and Bowlby);
- proposed the notion of social learning via reinforcement and conditioning (considered by Pavlov, Skinner and Bandura);
- highlighted the influence of culture, context and the environment (evident in socio-cultural theories and developmental frameworks, such as those of Vygostky, Bruner and Bronfenbrenner).

Essentially, the message we wish to disseminate in relation to the growth of developmental psychology is that while knowledge has increased in breadth, depth and sophistication, many of the issues raised and questions asked early in the twentieth century still remain current. It is unlikely there will ever be one specific theory that adequately explains how children grow and develop, but we should guard against 'throwing the baby out with the bathwater'. As is clearly highlighted by Sameroff (2010), in the argument for a unified theory of development that integrates behavioural change and socio-cultural context, central questions about the nature of children's development tend to go in and out of focus as new knowledge emerges. Our role as practitioners is to learn from each theory in relation to its strengths, and to ensure that we do not overlook the value of any weakness or criticism in moving our understanding forward. As the adage goes, the only real mistake we can make is one from which we learn nothing.

Theories of learning and development

Developmental psychology is concerned with describing and scientifically explaining physical and psychological change across the lifespan with a particular emphasis on theorising about why such change occurs (Bukatko & Daehler, 2011). A theory is an organised set of ideas that attempts to make sense of research findings such as experimental data or observations. Areas of development or developmental domains are often presented using the SPICE acronym, and include:

- Social development
- Physical development
- Intellectual development
- Communication and language development
- Emotional development.

Crucially, as well as being a means of describing and explaining behaviour, a theory can be used to predict behaviour in a given circumstance and should therefore be testable. Theories are useful in this sense because being able to predict the kinds of things that influence children's health and development means we are better able to plan effective policy and practice. Indeed, the very function of this book is to share theoretical ideas and research findings with a view to informing professional play practice. The following sections briefly explain some of the central theories of child development that have influenced practice. Some of these were discussed when considering theories of play in Chapter 1. Here we consider theories in relation to how they have contributed to our understanding of how children learn and develop more generally.

Sigmund Freud proposed a *psychosexual theory of development*. Although many of his ideas are often dismissed as outlandish, his contribution to developmental psychology cannot be underestimated. Firstly, he proposed that the mind is comprised of both conscious and unconscious elements (often presented using the iceberg metaphor) (see Figure 2.2). Secondly, Freud drew our attention to the important role early childhood experiences have in shaping development and personality; and thirdly, he introduced the notion of defence mechanisms as a means of coping with anxiety. According to Freud, only a small amount of the mind is conscious, holding immediate thoughts and experiences. The preconscious mind is like our general memory – we can selectively retrieve information from here, and information may be drawn into our conscious mind involuntarily too (e.g. by association). The largest part of the mind, however, is the unconscious, where Freud argued we used to get rid of information that caused pain or anxiety. He argued that information in the unconscious mind shaped behaviour but could only be accessed with considerable effort (e.g. with the support of a therapist). As presented in Chapter 1, Anna Freud and Melanie Klein were both influenced by these ideas, and we will return in Chapter 5 to the functions of specific value of particular play activities in their work.

Freud argued that development is shaped by two internal drives, thanatos (death/ aggression instinct) and libidos (instinct toward life and reproduction). He believed that there were three elements to our final personality, the Id, the Ego and the Superego. The Id can be defined as the pleasure-seeking or selfish part of the self, our need for self-

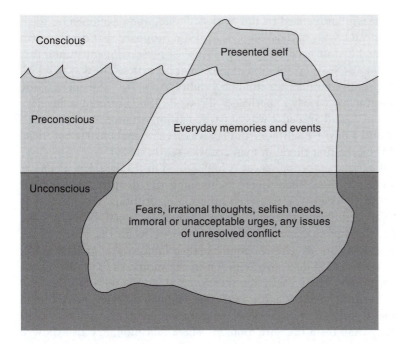

Figure 2.1 The iceberg metaphor of self based on the theory of Freud

satisfaction. The Superego is the moral or just part of the self, our understanding of how we ought to behave from an idealistic perspective. The Ego acts as a mediator between the two, the rational part of the self, which accepts the views of both the Id and the Superego and attempts to formulate a more realistic, compromise position. According to Freud, the Id is present from birth whereas the Ego and the Superego develop over time. Freud proposed that children had to negotiate particular psychosexual stages throughout childhood, at which time the pleasure-seeking energies of the Id would be focused on particular body zones (Oral, Anal, Phallic and Genital). The proposed significance of these and the importance of early parenting experiences can be found in any number of psychology texts, and there is neither scope nor need to discuss them here. Of importance is that any conflict between the Id, Ego and Superego is successfully resolved. To help ensure this, Freud proposed we employ a number of defence mechanisms, including:

- *denial* – pretending something isn't happening;
- *displacement* – taking out feelings on something or someone else;
- *intellectualisation* – focusing on the intellectual elements of a situation rather than having to deal with its emotional impact;
- *projection* – attributing negative thoughts or feelings to someone else;
- *regression* – returning to less mature behaviours in reaction to emotional events rather than developing a coping strategy (e.g. tantrums, crying);
- *repression* – unconsciously forgetting something due to anxiety;
- *suppression* – consciously trying to forget something if it makes you unhappy;
- *sublimation* – getting rid of desire in a socially acceptable way (e.g. physical exercise).

Erik Erikson was heavily influenced by the work of Freud, and developed his ideas further into a *psychosocial theory of development*. Erikson proposed that development of the self was motivated by our need to develop a sense of personal identity, and that this was achieved via the successful resolution of particular life crises. The way in which crises at each stage are resolved influences children's ability to resolve subsequent crises, highlighting the importance of early experiences. Erikson (1963) offered a developmental perspective on play, and argued it was of particular importance to developing a sense of competence and a positive self-esteem. Play was seen as particularly beneficial in the early years (during the first three lifespan crises) – see Table 2.1.

The importance of early social experiences is highlighted in the *attachment theory* of *John Bowlby*. In the 1940s, Rene Spitz documented the disturbing behaviour exhibited by babies and children who had been raised in institutions. Despite having had their basic needs met, the children demonstrated severe emotional difficulties and developmental delay. Bowlby suggested that these problems were the result of the children failing to develop secure attachment bonds. In their famous wire monkey study, Harlow and Zimmerman (1959) demonstrated that infant monkeys spent more time with a cloth-covered monkey than a wire monkey, even when the wire monkey had provided them with food. In times of emotional distress (such as being placed in an unfamiliar environment), the infant monkeys were also more inclined to seek comfort from the cloth monkey than from the wire monkey. The infant monkeys also showed more confidence in exploring a new environment when the cloth mother was present.

Bowlby (1969) suggested that this emotional connection was as important as nutrition, and that the way in which babies are biologically programmed to ensure the development of this emotional bond follows a particular sequence. In the first two months of life, babies display signalling behaviours such as crying and smiling, which draw the attention of the carer/s. At this early stage these behaviours are shown indiscriminately, but gradually (from 2 or 3 months onward) are used more frequently in the presence of the main carer/s, strengthening the developing bond. By 6 months attachment bonds have usually developed.

Using the strange situation technique, which involves evaluating how a baby reacts to being left alone with a stranger before being reunited with the caregiver, Ainsworth *et al.* (1978) identified particular attachment styles: secure, avoidant and ambivalent. Securely attached infants have experienced responsive and sensitive care and, just like the infant monkeys and the cloth model, are more confident in dealing with challenging situations. The role of these early relationships, often developed through playful interactions, is vital in shaping the brain, future emotional wellbeing and the way in which we deal with stress and anxiety (Gerhardt, 2004; Greenberg, 2006). This is closely related to the concept of resilience, and will be discussed further in Chapter 5.

Although Bowlby mainly considered mother–child relationships, equally important attachments are of course made with fathers. These may not necessarily be with biological parents and can be multiple (Dykas & Cassidy, 2011). Focusing on early relationships, Jennings (1999) usefully reminds us that problems not only arise through a child being under-held (owing to lack of warmth, security and appropriate stimulation) but also as a result of their being over-held (by being over-protected, prevented from taking risks or developing a sense of independence) and also distortedly-held (through physical abuse, neglect or sexual abuse). Research with children adjusting to life with

Table 2.1 Erikson's stages of the lifespan

Age (months)	Crises	Features	Play stage and focus
Birth–1	Trust v mistrust	Having trust that basic needs will be met, being able to depend on caregivers in predictable ways	AUTOCOSMIC play – physical and sensory, focused on developing an understanding of the bodily self, an important precursor to self-esteem
1–3	Autonomy v shame and doubt	Developing a gradual sense of independence, learning to manage and control behaviour	MICROSPHERIC play – the beginning of object play, learning to understand the impact of the self of the environment
3–6	Initiative v guilt	Having the confidence to explore and experiment. Being able to meet new challenges	MACROSPHERIC play – increasingly social play, role play and pretend play all lead to an understanding of other people's perspectives
6–12	Industry v inferiority	To function as a competent and confident learner	
12–20	Identity v role confusion	To understand one's place in the world, and role in the family, community and wider society	
20–40	Intimacy v isolation	To share the self with another in a reciprocal relationship	
40–65	Generativity v stagnation	Being productive, the need to nurture others or to have had an impact on the world, the need to feel we are making a difference	
65+	Integrity v despair	Being at peace with the self, accepting of achievements with no regret	

foster and adoptive parents demonstrates that attachment bonds can be established later than Bowlby originally anticipated, and can be rebuilt following trauma (Howe, 2006).

Ivan Pavlov founded the theory of *classical conditioning*. His work on the salivation reflex in dogs demonstrated that it was possible to pair an involuntary physiological response (e.g. salivation) with a neutral stimulus (e.g. the ringing of a bell). By presenting a trigger for the physiological response (e.g. food) alongside the neutral stimulus (e.g. the bell), eventually the bell alone could activate salivation.

In a procedure that would no longer be considered ethical practice, in their study of Little Albert, Watson and Rayner (1920) demonstrated how fear could be conditioned. Little Albert was given a white rat to play with, and initially he showed no fear of the animal; in fact he was happy to touch, stroke and lean toward it. In subsequent trials, each time the rat was presented, an iron bar was struck behind Albert, causing a startled fear response. Over time, the presentation of the rat without any striking of the iron bar produced a fear response on its own. This fear response was also generalised to things with similar characteristics such as a toy rabbit, white beard and cotton wool. The range of behaviours that can be explained in this way is not extensive, although understanding that children can learn in this way has proven useful for helping them to overcome anxiety and trauma, for example, in desensitisation therapy.

B. F. Skinner developed a further social learning theory called *operant conditioning*. Operant conditioning differs from classical conditioning in that it does not rely on the pairing of a physiological response. In operant conditioning, any two behaviours can be paired through reinforcement. Skinner famously taught pigeons to 'read' labelled levers by giving the reward of food when they performed the correct action. His theory had an important impact on behaviour modification and educational practices, for example, emphasising the importance of positive reinforcement over punishment. In essence, this theory suggests that a behaviour is more likely to be repeated if it is positively reinforced.

Albert Bandura developed *social learning theory*, which proposed that children learn through observation and imitation. In his classic 'bobo doll' study, Bandura (1973) demonstrated that when a child observed an adult behaving aggressively toward the inflatable doll, they were more likely to repeat this behaviour when left to play with the doll alone. Bandura also found that the influence of role models changed over time, beginning with primary caregivers and family members, to friends and peers and then others of significance such as teachers. It is very easy to think of examples of children learning in this way and, indeed, even young babies show their propensity toward imitation, mimicking the facial expressions of an adult at as early as 2 weeks (Meltzoff & Moore, 1999). Jennings (1999) also reminds us that children learn in this way from inappropriate role models and that behaviours exhibited may not always be positive. Bandura later extended his theory to consider the processes at work during social learning. His model of reciprocal determinism proposes four prerequisites for successful social learning: (1) attention – the child must attend to the behaviour being modelled; (2) retention – the behaviour must be remembered; (3) reproduction – the behaviour is recalled and the child has the skills necessary to reproduce it; and (4) motivation – the child is motivated by reinforcement (as in Skinner's theory of operant conditioning) to reproduce the action.

The theories presented so far all suggest the child is relatively passive, with development simply happening without them consciously engaging in the process. *Jean Piaget*, however, in his *constructivist theory of cognitive development* attributed the child an active role in their learning. Piaget was particularly interested in children's logic and was influenced by Darwin's theory of evolution, which proposed that organisms grew in complexity in order to adapt to their environment. Piaget proposed that learning and development are motivated by a drive toward equilibrium, the need for information stored in our minds to accurately reflect what we understand about the world. In order to achieve equilibrium we have two mechanisms of change, namely assimilation and accommodation. We use these mechanisms to house information correctly, to add to our existing schema (pockets of knowledge) or to amend them. Adding information to an existing schema involves assimilation while amending a schema requires accommodation.

Key developmental tasks in relation to children's development from a Piagetian perspective are: gaining object permanence (knowing something exists when it is out of sight); a move away from egocentricism (understanding another person's perspective); symbolic thought (enabling one object to represent another); conservation (understanding constant object properties regardless of presentation); and abstract or hypothetical thought (being able to consider things not yet experienced). Piaget is perhaps most well known for his proposition that development occurs in stages (ages are approximate) (see Table 2.2). His description of how play develops is aligned to both these stages and dependent on achieving key developmental tasks. For Piaget, children learned best when they engaged in first-hand experience.

Lev Vygostky also proposed an active role for the child in his *social constructivist* theory of development. He proposed that rather than learning through self-guided exploration, children's skills and abilities were cultivated by social interaction. Rather than being biologically driven, development was culturally specific and co-constructed. He proposed that children were motivated to learn by their need to communicate and become socially accepted. Whereas Piaget saw language as a product of thought, Vygostky proposed language was a tool for thought, in which initially thinking would be done out loud before finally becoming internalised. A key element of Vygostky's theory was the zone of proximal development. This, he argued, represented the difference between what a child could achieve alone and what they could achieve with assistance. This argument heavily influenced early years teaching practice and the view that children's learning was best supported through sensitive interactions. However, it is important to note that Vygostky (1978) believed that play promoted higher-level thinking, 'as though the child was a head taller than themselves' (p. 102). He proposed that imaginative play, in particular, freed children from the constraints of reality, enabling them to safely try on roles and try out ideas.

Increased communication skills and opportunity for social interaction are also the motivating forces behind the patterns of social development observed by *Margaret Parten* in her *developmental approach to social play*. Parten (1932) suggests six stages of play:

1. *unoccupied behaviour* – not playing, simply observing;
2. *solitary play* – child plays alone, uninterested in others;

**Table 2.2 Piaget's stages of development,
key characteristics and associated play types**

Stages of development	Characteristics	Associated play types
Sensorimotor period (birth–2 years)	Learning and exploration involves the senses, with a move from involuntary reflex action to controlled action and an increasing emphasis on cause and effect. Object permanence develops at around 8 months	Practice play Sensory activity, often repetitive
Pre-operational period (2–7 years)	Increasingly complex logic, a period of intense development, child begins to use internal images, symbols and language. A move away from geocentricism occurs at around 4 years	Symbolic play Small world play Symbolic play Role play Art and drawing Simple rule-based games (although rules may be treated flexibly)
Concrete operational (7–11 years)	Can conserve and mentally arrange objects Beginnings of understanding	Games with rules Increasingly complex
Formal operational (11+ years)	Can weigh up alternatives and consider the outcomes of hypothetical scenarios	Games with rules Increasingly complex Playing with ideas and roles

3. *onlooker behaviour* – child watches the play of others and may talk to the children involved but this talk does not relate to the play;
4. *parallel play* – plays alongside others, often imitating what is being played nearby but with no interaction;
5. *associative play* – the children appear to be playing together but their activities are not organised;
6. *co-operative play* – playing together in more organised activities where they share intentions about the progress of the play.

As described in Chapter 1, the work of Piaget and Vygostky was synthesised by *Jerome Bruner* in his *cognitive developmental theory*. Bruner (1974) proposed that children learn via three modes of representation: enactive representation (action-based), iconic representation (image-based), and symbolic representation (language-based). These are sequential, with one mode merging into the next. The nature and success of children's development was strongly related to the learning environment and social experience.

The significance of the wider society for children's learning and development has been captured in *Bronfenbrenner's ecological systems* approach. Urie Bronfenbrenner (1979[PD3]) places the child at the centre of the larger socio-cultural context, surrounded by a series of external contexts that can directly or indirectly shape behaviour:

- *the micro-system* – the immediate environments in which the child is operating;
- *the meso-system* – the influence of two or more micro-systems interacting with one another;
- *the exo-system* – environments where the child is not directly involved but where there is potential for them to influence their life experiences;
- *the macro-system* – the larger cultural or societal context;
- *the chrono-system* – the influence of history and time.

This is not a theory as such because it is almost impossible to test (owing to its intricacy), but it reminds us that while children may learn in the ways theorists suggest, it is important for us to appreciate that development occurs in a wider context. The way in which difference and diversity can influence play and development is considered in Chapter 6.

Having a broad understanding of the various ways that children learn and develop is important to our practice. Theories and research evidence tell us that:

- Secure, warm and loving relationships are vitally important to children's health and development.
- Early experiences can influence the course of development across domains (in ways that we can see but potentially in ways that we cannot see).
- Children learn through imitation, modelling and by association.
- Sensory and physical experiences underpin much of children's development (children must learn about the physical self before they develop identity and self-esteem).
- Children learn through self-directed experiences as well through activities where they are offered sensitive support.
- Learning requires children's attention, enthusiasm and motivation.
- Emotional health, self-esteem and a sense of independence play an important role in development.
- Children's development must be viewed in social and cultural context.
- Play becomes more social and cognitively complex over time.

See Figure 2.2 for a summary of an ecological systems model of development.

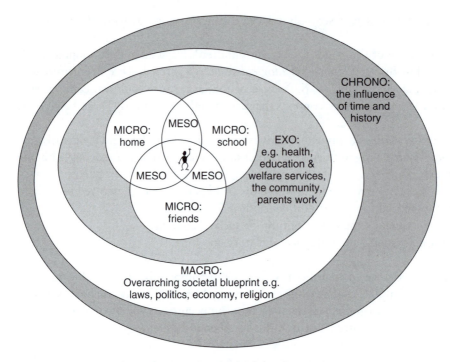

Figure 2.2 An ecological systems model of development

An outline of children's development and play behaviour from birth to adolescence

There is not scope to consider children's development from birth to adolescence comprehensively in this book (if you would like to read a detailed account, see Sheridan, Howard & Alderson, 2011). Here, however, we will present some of children's main developmental milestones and play behaviours from birth through to early adolescence.

0–6 months

- *Social* – interaction mainly involves primary caregiver/s and family members.
- *Physical* – gradual progression from involuntary movements toward controlled actions; develops hand grasp and can co-ordinate movement of objects to the mouth for exploration.
- *Intellectual* – starts to understand the permanence of people but not things.
- *Communication* – cries for immediate attention, also uses gaze, body movements and vocalisation during interactions.
- *Emotional* – develops strong emotional bond with primary caregiver/s.

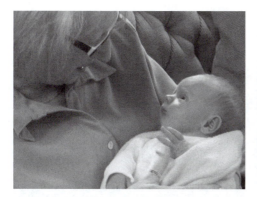

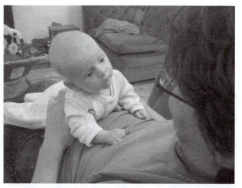

a) Just days after birth, this newborn gazes up at his grandmother, the beginning of their bonding process

b) A couple of months later, he is able to lift his head, and can gain and maintain the attention of his Dad

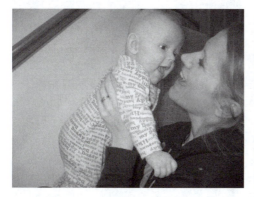

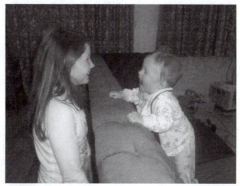

c) A little less delicate at 5 months, he delights in some physical play and the sustained attention of his Mum

d) Nearing 6 months, peek-a-boo with his sister becomes one of this baby's favourite games

Play at 0–6 months involves exploration of the body and senses. Objects will be brought to the mouth for exploration, sound can be made by shaking or banging. Baby will enjoy experiencing new sights, sounds and textures. Actions may often be repetitive. Important here is the development of strong emotional bonds with primary caregivers, and baby will enjoy the eye contact, interaction and attention afforded by rhymes, singing or peek-a-boo.

6–12 months

- *Social* – baby continues to enjoy interaction with primary caregiver/s and family members during play; interest in interacting with other familiar children and adults may also emerge.

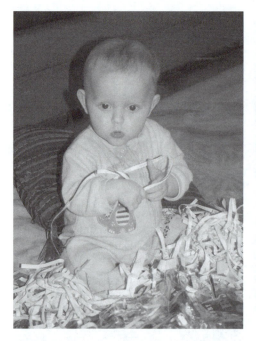

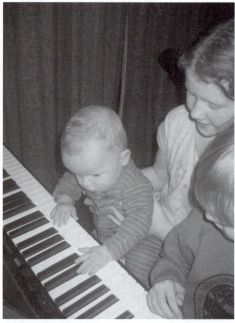

a) At 7 months, baby can sit and grasp nearby objects. He enjoys the sound and feel of this shredded paper

b) He has increased control over his movements now and with his siblings baby enjoys the noise he can make by banging his hands onto the piano keys

c) At 8 months, the light reflecting on this shiny ribbon and wrapping paper sustains his attention for much longer than the present itself!

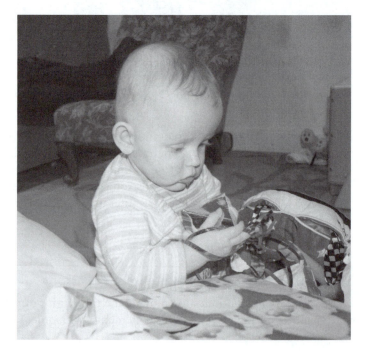

- *Physical* – well-developed reach and grasp, and can obtain nearby objects. Can pass objects from hand to hand and bang items together. Gradually develops ability to release items from hands, to roll over, sit and crawl.
- *Intellectual* – develops object permanence and knows items exist when they are removed from sight; begins to imitate actions, begins to understand cause and effect.
- *Communication* – a wider range of nonverbal signals and vocalisations may be used to indicate wants and needs. Comprehends a few single words.
- *Emotional* – secure attachment bond with primary caregiver/s means baby becomes more able to tolerate being alone for short periods; baby may develop an emotional bond with a particular toy for security.

Play at 6–12 months still largely involves the senses, and baby enjoys being able to reach for and manipulate objects. Becomes more able to explore through being able to sit up and perhaps move around. They will continue to enjoy rattling, banging and sliding objects. With a secure emotional bond they are confident to explore their environment but need to know their caregiver is proximal. Baby may become attached to a particular toy for comfort and security here (often called a transitional object).

12–18 months

- *Social* – becomes interested in watching the activities of others but is self-oriented. By the end of this stage, children may begin to play with others.
- *Physical* – increased mobility (cruising and walking), improved co-ordination, balance and muscle tone, drive toward exploration of physical capabilities.
- *Intellectual* – understands cause and effect, imitates readily and can recall actions to imitate from memory; may begin to attach meaning and names to objects; less repetition and more interest in object details.
- *Communication* – first words emerge, with a growing interest in using language to signify needs; control over the voice motivates tuneful vocalisations and self-talk. The first two-word utterances are produced by the end of this stage.
- *Emotional* – may become frustrated at not being able to always get their own way or have all of the things in their surroundings for themselves, as does not yet recognise other points of view.

Play at 12–18 months still largely involves physical movement and the senses, although an emerging appreciation of cause and effect means items that involve push, pull or simple button pressing are particularly inviting. They may become interested in mark-making and exploring the finer properties of objects, such as putting things in and out of containers and stacking (as well as knocking down!). May engage in imitative play involving familiar items (such as a bottle or toothbrush), with dolls or soft toys. Particularly important here is that the child is supported in gaining control over their actions, understanding consequence and developing their independence.

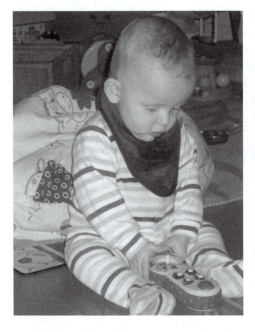

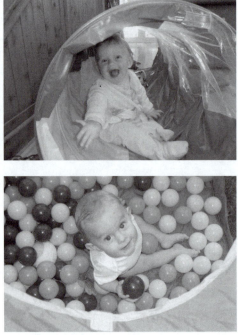

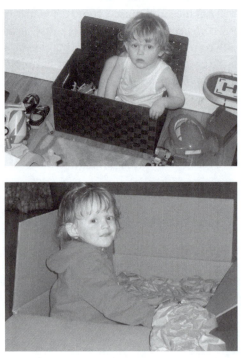

a) At 12 months, baby can now press the buttons on this electronic phone

b, c) Being able to crawl means there are many more places to explore

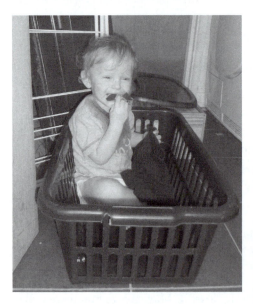

d, e, f) At 18 months, he enjoys climbing in and out of boxes, finding out about his size and testing out his physical abilities. This fascination continues for many months!

18–24 months

- *Social* – may begin to engage in parallel activity.
- *Physical* – gross motor skills improve; gains confidence in running, climbing and carrying items, exploring body size and capabilities; fine motor skills allow manipulation of small objects.
- *Intellectual* – sense of danger is limited, and child remains relatively egocentric although simple pretence may start to emerge; actively builds memories of events

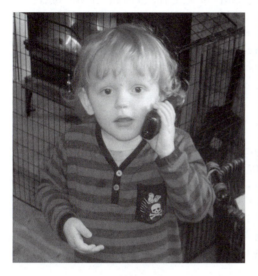

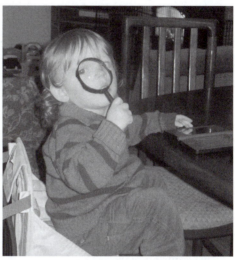

a) At 19 months, baby imitates what he sees others doing around the house, and clearly knows how to use the telephone

b) He has only seen a magnifying glass being used on the television but, surprisingly, he imitates the correct action

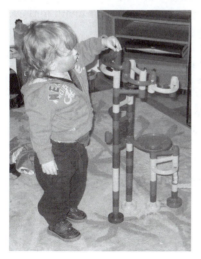

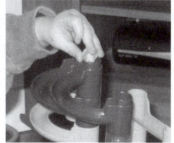

c) His brother has built this marble tower, but he can place and let go of the marbles well and he enjoys watching them spiral down (note the development of his pincer grip) and recognises patterns and sequences, for example, in stories and rhymes; increased concentration span.

- *Communication* – growth in language skill and level of vocabulary; two-word utterances and gestures used effectively for communication.
- *Emotional* – keen to show likes and dislikes, growing independence.

Play at 18–24 months play becomes more intricate and complex. The child may engage more frequently in small world play, showing in this play that they know what things are and what they normally do. Emphasis is on the realistic use of objects, however. They are particularly interested in imitation and copying the actions of others. There may be simple role play at familiar situations (e.g. mum feeding baby). Becoming aware of relative size, they may explore boxes or other play equipment. They show a growing interest in mark-making. Of importance here is supporting the growth of social skill and encouraging parallel play and simple interactions with other children.

2–3 years

- *Social* – becomes more confident in social situations and may engage in parallel play more frequently; solitary play remains predominant but child may start to try out some simple social interaction and turn-taking skills.
- *Physical* – continued growth in physical capabilities; may like to kick a ball, roll, jump, skip or hop; can hold and direct pencils or crayons more easily now.
- *Intellectual* – can substitute one thing for another (symbolic thought); begins to match colours and shapes; memory, recall and sequencing may be evident in scripts used during play.
- *Communication* – will try out a wider range of language and sounds with growing confidence; begins to rely less on nonverbal means of communication.
- *Emotional* – some evidence of understanding others' feelings and perspectives but self-space remains important; trying out new social skills needs encouragement from caregivers; the transitional object may become important once again in these unfamiliar situations. Children begin to develop gender identity.

Play at 2–3 years gradually involves more and more pretence. The ability to allow one thing to stand for another opens up a range of new play opportunities, and children may start to pretend at situations that they are aware of but have not necessarily experienced (shops, library or post office). Simple puzzles can be completed, and children may have a particular interest in drawing and copying marks. They may show some awareness of others' feelings and ideas (tentatively offering another a child a toy on their request), but will still show frustration that others do not automatically understand (or abide by!) their thoughts and wishes. Ensuring the maintenance of a positive sense of self in unfamiliar social situations is important here.

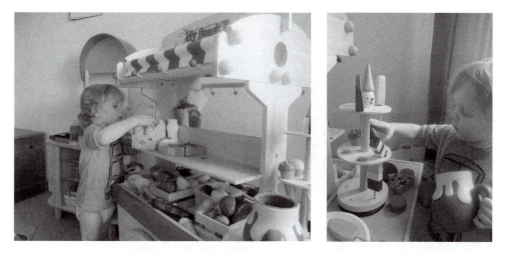

a) At 2 years old, this little one spends half an hour or more playing shop; b) Even though playing alone, his play involves lots of vocalisation and self 'talk'. He gets quite frustrated at trying to balance these ice creams in their holder!

3–5 years

- *Social* – engages in associative and gradually co-operative play; may return to onlooker, solitary or parallel activity in new or unfamiliar situations; may show some signs of friendship behaviours with frequent playmates.
- *Physical* – increasing skill in gross motor co-ordination and balance; fine motor skills also develop, for example, in drawing, cutting out or using a knife and fork.
- *Intellectual* – sequencing abilities develop; shows ability to use knowledge from one situation in another; concentration span markedly improves; shows clear awareness of real and pretend.
- *Communication* – language skills allow more lengthy and meaningful communication, which is no longer predominantly related to requests, and children will enjoy asking what and why questions. Interest may grow in making music; understanding of the language rules is evident in children's play with words and their meaning. Different voices may be used in role play.
- *Emotional* – new social situations place new demands on the child. Children must learn to negotiate roles and rules in social groups, to share and take turns. Children begin to develop empathy for another's feelings.

Play at 3–5 years comprises a full repertoire of sensory and physical activity, small world play and role play as well as drawing and art. The process of making or drawing is more important than the final product, however, and children may not know (or be able to name) what they are drawing until it is complete. They may enjoy hearing and making music. Scripts in play may become more elaborate and imaginative. Play becomes more social, although a particular challenge here is learning how to manage

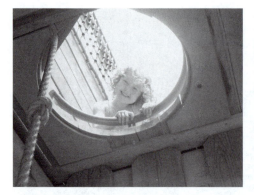

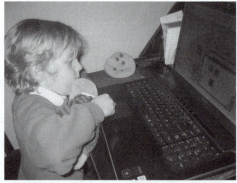

a) This 3-year-old is very proud of climbing to the top of this climbing frame and enjoys peeking down at the ground far below

b) Just starting school, this 4-year-old already has a keen interest in computer play (and teddy joins in too!)

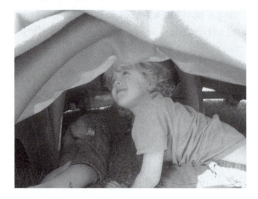

c) This makeshift den provides hours of building and hiding fun

these situations in terms of turn-taking, negotiation and group rules while at the same time seeking social acceptance.

5–7 years

- *Social* – social skills continue to increase, and group acceptance becomes more important; there is an increase in real co-operative activity; more friendships may be made and no longer rely on immediate play situations.
- *Physical* – children have a well-developed sense of their physical capabilities and may begin to enjoy group new sports that extend their skills; they enjoy physical risk and challenge.
- *Intellectual* – there is a growing appreciation of rules, although these are often treated flexibly; a personal style may develop in drawings.
- *Communication* – further understanding about the rules of language becomes evident in children's enjoyment of increasingly complex humour and jokes.

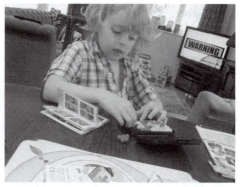

b) At 6 years, he becomes more interested in copying patterns

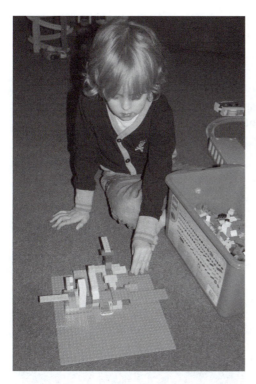

a) Aged 5, this little boy enjoys building Lego-brick models of his own design

- *Emotional* – with a secure base children are confident to meet the many new challenges they may face in the school and other contexts to which they may now be exposed.

Play at 5–7 years reflects children's growing appreciation of rules. Board games and made-up group games may be of particular interest (although they may still wish to bend these rules at times!). They enjoy making things from models or from their own imagination. Preference toward particular social groups or particular activities may become apparent.

7–11 years

- *Social* – friends become more stable, and children may enjoy arranging to meet up outside of the school environment.
- *Physical* – children continue to delight in the physical capabilities of their bodies, testing balance or co-ordination through gymnastics or dance. The bodies of girls may begin to change toward the end of this period as they move closer to puberty.

- *Intellectual* – sophisticated understanding of rules; are able to conserve volume, mass and length. Can mentally arrange items by size, weight or height; can solve concrete problems.
- *Communication* – children may begin to use alternative forms of communication such as mobile phones and networking sites. These require them to develop a new vocabulary. They may also begin to test the boundaries of what is appropriate or inappropriate in general and in different social contexts.

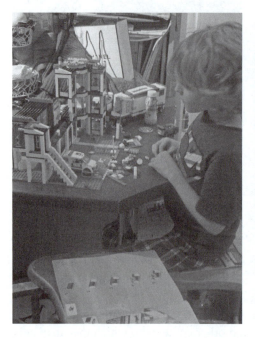

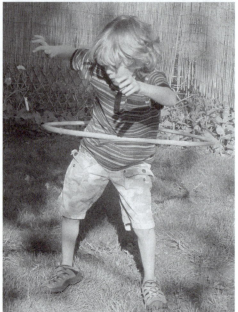

a) At nearly 7 years, this little boy really enjoys following the instructions for complex Lego models

b) The same child also shows complex physical abilities and, much to his older sister's dismay, he beats her in a hula-hoop challenge, managing over a hundred gyrations!

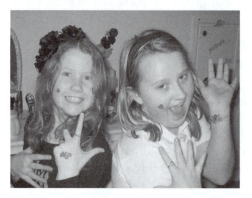

c) Nearing 11 years, these friends spend many hours trying out new hairstyles and make-up techniques, beginning to play with their identities

- *Emotional* – children must manage friendships alongside growing educational demands; children may be exposed to hurtful situations, for example, when friendships are broken, when they are not able to join a social group or when others make comments about them.

Play at 7–11 years is likely to involve more group-based games with increasingly complex rules. There may be increased electronic play, for example, with computers, game stations or handheld consoles. Children may enjoy writing stories, creative activities on a large or small scale as well as dance and drama. Personal preferences and hobbies may become increasingly apparent.

11 years onwards

- *Social* – children become aware of the views of others and reflect on their sense of self in light of these views.
- *Physical* – puberty brings great physical change for both girls and boys.
- *Intellectual* – children are able to think in abstract or hypothetical ways; they can weigh up alternatives and the consequences of particular actions.
- *Communication* – may return to questioning everything as they struggle to reconcile what ought to be with what actually is.
- *Emotional* – physical change is likely to bring about emotional anxiety; children may become oppositional as they test boundaries and reflect on their sense of self.

Play at 11 years onward may involve hanging out with friends, social networking or online gaming. Young people may continue to enjoy hobbies and sports. They play at real life in cooking or rearranging their rooms. Young people often play with their identities through changing their image or their attitude toward certain things as they try to understand their place in the world, the family, the community and wider society.

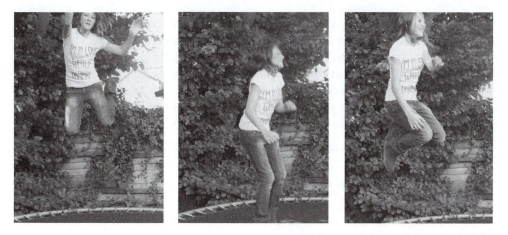

a, b and c) At 13 years this young person still shows a real sense of enjoyment on the trampoline

Conclusion

Play offers children opportunities for learning and development across domains. From a social and emotional perspective, children have the opportunity to learn about themselves and others. They learn about the impact their behaviour has in social situations, developing the ability to resolve conflict and make friends. In play children can *try out* different ways of dealing with social situations and *try on* feelings, emotions and social roles with minimal consequence. From a cognitive perspective, play offers opportunities to learn about objects, concepts and ideas and to develop problem-solving strategies. The emergence of symbolic thought enables them to use one thing to stand for something else (for example, in pretend play), which is an important precursor to more complex ways of thinking. Play offers opportunities for the development of language and communication skills, for example, learning new vocabulary, the way that words are pronounced as well as how they can be used in different ways. Play involves gross and fine motor movements and as such promotes co-ordination and physical health. The role of early physical experiences influences the development of the vestibular system, which can impact on learning and development in a variety of ways (Goddard-Blythe, 2004).

As we have seen in this chapter, however, children learn in a number of different ways. Of importance to this text is demonstrating how play is particularly valuable for maximising what children learn, enhancing their development across domains by making the learning mechanisms we have discussed in this chapter more effective. We propose that this relies on us considering children's perceptions of what it means to play, understanding the kinds of things that facilitate a sense of playfulness. The following chapter will consider this issue. Particularly valuable characteristics of play are also discussed in Chapter 5 when assessing the play environment.

Now that you have read the chapter

- In your practice, make observational notes about when you think a child has learned something in each of the different ways described in this chapter.
- See if you are able to observe children exhibiting any of the characteristics associated with Piaget's stages of development (e.g. egocentricism).
- Make some observations of different-aged children at play (what they are playing, where, who with?). Are your observations congruent with what you have read in this chapter? If not, why might this be?

Useful further reading

Gerhardt, S. (2004) *Why Love Matters: How Affection Shapes a Baby's Brain* (London: Routledge).
A well-evidenced, coherent and accessible text, which provides an excellent account of the significance of early relationships for children's development.

3 Playfulness

Aims of the chapter

- To differentiate between the observable act of play and the state of playfulness.
- To identify how playfulness may be the key ingredient in children's play.
- To argue that playfulness may be the basis of a shared understanding about play between different play practitioners.
- To argue that by understanding children's perceptions of play, play practitioners may gain insight into the state of playfulness.
- To describe a methodology that enables play practitioners to identify children's perceptions of play.

Introduction

As discussed in Chapters 1 and 2, there is a range of play theories underpinning play practice, and different play practices will draw on different theories. However, irrespective of professional play background and theoretical understanding, all play practitioners share an intuitive belief that play benefits children. When observing children at play it is possible to see that they are happy, physically active, socialising with other children, practising skills and problem-solving, all of which are beneficial for children's development. However, how do we know that children are actually developing these skills and attributes; what is the evidence? Unfortunately, although growing, empirical evidence for the benefits of play is scarce. As Lester and Russell (2008) state: 'many studies of play remain controversial, contradictory and often lack empirical support' (p. 37). This lack of evidence is constant across the different play practices and, certainly within early years educational practice, has led to the 'idealisation of play' (Sutton-Smith & Kelly-Byrne, 1984).

In this chapter it will be argued that the lack of empirical evidence arises from differences in defining the observable act of play as well as the more accepted methodological and experimental weaknesses inherent within play studies (e.g. Smith, 2010; Smith & Whitney, 1987). It will be also be argued that, rather than focusing on the observable act of play, which is problematic, practitioners should focus on playfulness and that it is this that is ultimately beneficial for children. In order to understand playfulness, and in keeping with current beliefs about children and childhood, it will be suggested that the voice of children should be sought and that play practice should be based on children's definitions of play, which encompasses playfulness. A rigorous and usable methodology will be presented, which will enable play practitioners to elicit children's views of play.

Defining play

As discussed in Chapter 1, there are different ways to define play; in part these are dependent upon practice background, and often ways of defining play are overlapping. As a starting point it is probably useful to state what play is not, and the exploratory behaviour that very young children, and those new to an activity, engage in is different from play.

A clear distinction between play and exploration was made by C. Hutt (1976), who looked at the exploratory behaviour elicited in children when presented with a novel object. She concluded that in this situation children exhibited two types of behaviour. Initially, children were completely focused on the object, engaging in concentrated behaviour characterised by an intent facial expression. Over time this changed, with children less focused on the object and becoming more relaxed in their behaviour. The former she called 'exploratory behaviour', the latter she called 'play', with children moving from asking '"what does this object do?' to 'what can I do with this object?'" (p. 211). These two types of behaviour can be distinguished physiologically by heart rate variability, with a calm heart rate during play denoting a relaxed state and a variable heart rate during exploration denoting an attentive state (S. J. Hutt, Tyler, Hutt & Christopherson, 1989).

So, what is play? Traditionally, there have been three main ways to define play: by category, criteria or continuum (Howard, 2002). Piaget (1951) first proposed a categorical definition of play, defining it according to developmental stages of play aligned to his developmental stages of intellectual development. These play categories were: practice play, symbolic play and games with rules. However, these categories were criticised as children do not progress through distinct stages in their play, and the categories do not account for all types of play, for example, rough and tumble play. Smilansky (1968) developed this work and proposed a fourth category of constructive play, but, as Smith, Takhvar, Gore and Vollstedt (1986) point out, Piaget saw play as assimilative whereas constructive play is accommodative, and therefore does not fit this hierarchy.

Criteria or continuum definitions of play focus on behaviours and dispositions of play. A number of different criteria definitions have been proposed (e.g. Krasnor &

Pepler, 1980; Neumann, 1971; Rubin, Fein & Vandenberg, 1983), and suggested criteria include: locus of control (freedom to choose), intrinsic motivation (self-motivation to engage and stay with an activity), non-literality (displaying pretence) and positive affect (having fun). Using these criteria, an onlooker can determine whether an activity is play or not. Pellegrini (1991) developed this idea further to propose a continuum of play, with pure play defined when all criteria are used and less play-like activities using fewer criteria. Another way of defining play is by using play types founded on the different behaviours children display when playing (e.g. Hughes, 2006). What these different definitions have in common is that they are all based on theorists or adults looking at the observable act of play – it is an adult-led definition of play based on what is seen, and what is seen and ultimately understood as play may vary across different adult observers.

There are those who say that play cannot be defined (e.g. Moyles, 1989), as it is such an elusive concept and means different things to different people. Conversely, there are those who argue that because it is such an elusive concept that anything can be called play (Stallibrass, 1977). While both of these viewpoints are understandable, it is ultimately unhelpful for those attempting to provide empirical evidence for the benefits of play for children's development. There are also those who avoid defining play by discussing the creation of conditions, or a context, for children to play and those who identify play as a process. Facilitating the conditions or a context to enable children to play is shared by many play practitioners, especially the idea of a 'playful space' and the absence of adult direction within the play space enabling children to play freely (e.g. Brown, 2008; Winnicott, 1971). Likewise the notion of play as a process is one that is shared by many play practitioners. Within recreational play practice it often thought of as a cycle of activity with shared signals, which must be responded to in order to maintain the play behaviour (Sturrock & Else, 1998), whereas within educational play practice, play is often seen as an integrating mechanism bringing aspects of development together (Bruce, 2011). While these ideas are important and broaden our understanding of play, they remain adult-led understandings of play and do not help us evidence the benefits of play for children.

Playfulness

It has been argued that it is the internal, affective qualities of play that are important therapeutically and for development, such as: enthusiasm, motivation and willingness to engage (Moyles, 1989; Rogers & Sluss, 1999) and that these are different from the act of play. Dewey (1933) was the first to make the distinction between play and playfulness, arguing that playfulness was more important than play. He stated that, 'the former is an attitude of mind; the latter is an outward manifestation of this attitude' (p. 210). Another term for this might be 'disposition', as defined by Katz (1993) and Parker-Rees (1999), as a habit of mind or a characteristic way of responding to a situation. This playful attitude or disposition is seen as one of freedom, and this also accords with the 'flow state' identified by Csikszentmihalyi (1988, 1990), which is also characterised by internal affective qualities of pleasure, involvement and deep concentration. In psychoanalysis, Winnicott (1971) discusses the importance of the playful therapist and the playful patient in creating a playful space for the patient to develop and grow.

It would seem that all the above theorists are making a similar case for playfulness: that it is an attitude of mind that affects the approach taken to an activity, and it may be argued that this way of viewing playfulness rather than the play act itself may be the most helpful to play practitioners.

It is important to distinguish between the two interpretations of playfulness that exist within the literature. One is that playfulness is a personality trait of the individual (e.g. Lieberman, 1977; Singer & Singer, 1980), and the other is that it is a style, approach or attitude to an activity as discussed above. It is generally assumed that the personality trait of playfulness is static over time and independent of the environment, and as such this is not helpful to practitioners. Recent work from the field of occupational therapy on the state of playfulness has shown that playfulness may be viewed on a continuum of being more or less playful, and that this is dependent on time and space (e.g. Bronson & Bundy, 2001; Hamm, 2006). This is helpful to play practitioners, and how they might facilitate playfulness will be explored further in the chapters on the adult role and the environment.

Viewing the state of playfulness as a manifestation of different internal and affective qualities of play means that it is not as open to adult observation as the act of playing. We cannot assume that because a child is engaged in what looks like a play act that they are feeling playful. Consider the Scenarios A and B below.

Scenario A

It is planning time in a reception class. A girl sits at a table where a variety of puzzles are laid out for the children to complete. She chooses a number puzzle and becomes engrossed in completing the puzzle. Occasionally she shares a comment and laughs with the other children who are also completing puzzles at the table.

Scenario B

It is planning time in a reception class. A girl goes to the cupboard and chooses a number puzzle. She sits on the floor and becomes engrossed in completing the puzzle. She doesn't look up or talk to the other children around her who are engaged in various activities including completing puzzles.

Both of these scenarios look very similar and look like play, but when shown photographs of the different scenarios adult observers consistently say that both scenarios are play and the children are playing. When children are shown photographs of the different scenarios children consistently say that the first scenario is not play and therefore they are not feeling playful, while in the second scenario they are playing and feel playful. So, to understand playfulness play practitioners need to go beyond what they see and talk to children about what is play.

Children's perceptions of play

Asking children about their views of play and playing accords with current views of the child as being or being and becoming rather than just becoming, as discussed in Chapter 1. It is enabling children's voices to be heard and placing them at the heart of play, something that has been frequently overlooked in the play literature and by play practitioners despite calls to consider children's definitions of play (Wood & Attfield, 2005).

Historically, there has been a view that children do not distinguish between play and work (Isaacs, 1929; Manning & Sharp, 1977), and consequently there have been few attempts to elicit their views. However, research that has been conducted on children's perceptions of play has shown that children do distinguish between play and not play activities, and the environment they experience influences this. Although it may be argued that the majority of studies undertaken have been conducted in classroom environments where play and work are commonly held notions by educators, thereby influencing children's perceptions, it has been found that children make these same distinctions in the home (Holmes, 1999).

Research by King (1979) found that children described play activities as those that were voluntary, fun, under the child's control and did not involve adults. Conversely, work activities were described as those that were compulsory, under adult control and the adult was involved. Rothlein and Brett (1987) found that certain activities could be defined as play such as outside play and certain toys. Karrby (1989) showed that play activities could include pretence but didn't have to and involved rules set by children, whereas not play activities were taught activities, involved specific goals and sitting down. This study also identified that play definitions were dependent upon the setting children experienced, with children in more play-based, child-initiated settings identifying more activities as play. Children in more structured settings displayed a clearer distinction, with teacher-directed activities being described as not play and child-initiated activities as play.

Robson (1993), Wing (1995) and Keating *et al.* (2000) all conducted studies showing that a greater range of activities could be defined as play and not play, with an emphasis on child control determining play activities and adult control determining not play activities. Also, some activities could be identified on a continuum, with Robson (1993) identifying painting as not play and Wing (1995) showing it as play. This was also found in the Keating *et al.* (2000) study. Interestingly, there was ambiguity between the studies as to whether an activity had to be fun to be perceived as play, with some studies showing that it did whereas other studies showed that an activity did not have to be fun to be perceived as play.

All of the above methods used observational and interview methodology, which can be problematic with young children. Young children often have limited linguistic abilities, and it can be difficult for them to get their meaning across and for adults to understand them. It involves sustained concentration and a high cognitive load for children to interpret questions, recall activities and talk about them. There is often an issue concerned with power relations between young children and adults, with children saying what they think adults want to hear. Group interviews are often thought to be preferable to individual interviews with young children, as this overcomes the issue of power relations and children can encourage one another to speak. However, it may mean that not all children get to speak or the most vocal child influences the others in the group (Brooker, 2001; Westcott & Littleton, 2005). These difficulties have led to the development of a more child-friendly and systematic methodology to collect children's views about play.

The Activity Apperception Story Procedure (AASP)

The AASP (Howard, 2002) is a game-like, photographic categorisation method that is easy to use and child-friendly. It is a two-part procedure, which firstly requires children to post photographic stimuli into letter boxes labelled play or not play. Photographs of classroom activities are used rather than pictures as for young children these capture reality better than pictures (Kose, Beilin & O'Connor, 1983), and children respond well to the game-like procedure (Sturgess & Ziviani, 1996). The photographs depict a variety of classroom scenarios and are paired according to cues based on the previous studies of children's perceptions of play. These include: positive affect (whether an activity is fun or serious), space and constraint (whether an activity occurs at a table or on the floor), adult presence (present or not present) and type of activity (play or academic materials). Assessment of reliability is possible through repetition of the activity. The second part is a justification exercise requiring children to discuss their choices for a smaller number of photographs. A further study using this procedure also included the cue of social grouping (solitary, paired or group activity) (Howard, Jenvey & Hill, 2006).

The AASP procedure has also been applied using photographs of children's actual environments rather than staged scenarios (Howard & Westcott, 2007; Howard, Miles & Parker, 2008; Parker, 2008). This means that the cues contained within the photographic stimuli are developed further and the process is now known as the Revised Apperception Procedure (RAP). This means that the cues contained within the photographic stimuli are of the children's actual teachers, peers and equipment, thus making them more meaningful. In addition, a further cue has been investigated, that of choice, and it has been found that children perceive an activity as play when they have choice.

Studies using the AASP procedure have shown that children use the cues of teacher presence, space and constraint, positive affect, activity type and choice to differentiate between play and not play. Play is a more likely response if an activity does not involve adult presence, occurs on the floor, where positive affect is shown, and where the activity involves play-like rather than academic materials. The study involving social context identified cooperative and group activities as more play-like, and findings consistently demonstrate that children need to have choice to distinguish an activity as play. In addition, the findings also confirm that children's play and not play choices are dependent upon the type of setting experienced. Children appear to learn which cues are associated with play and not play activity. Children in less structured settings with higher levels of free play make fewer play and not play distinctions compared to children who have experienced a setting where there is a strong contrast between play and formal activities. In settings where adults frequently engaged with children in their play, photographs where an adult was present are still defined by children as play, suggesting that they accept them as play partners.

Overall, it can be seen that children are able to distinguish between play and not play-like activities and that their perceptions of play, while similar to those of adults, are also different (see Table 3.1). For example, adults do not consider the location of an activity when observing children at play nor do they consider the choice a child has in an activity. In addition, children's perceptions of play are also dependent upon experience, a finding not considered by the research looking at adult definitions of play. There is also the finding that children perceive play and not play activities on a continuum, with different activities being more or less like play. Recent research indicates that these cues are also used by older children who experience the Welsh Foundation Phase, a play-based curriculum that continues up to age 7 (Chapman, 2011; Owen-Leeds, 2012).

Children's perceptions of play and playfulness

So, if practitioners understand children's perceptions of play does this help in terms of understanding and utilising playfulness in practice? Current and ongoing research would suggest it does (McInnes, Howard, Miles & Crowley, 2009; Thomas, Howard

Table 3.1 Summary of cues used by children to characterise play

Cue	More like play	Less like play
Location	Floor	Table
Choice	Choice	No choice
Locus of control	Control with the child	Control with the adult
Adult presence	Adult not present	Adult present
Positive affect	Positive affect	Lack of positive affect
Activity type	Play-like	Work-like
Social grouping	Cooperative, group	Solitary
Adult evaluation	No adult evaluation	Adult evaluation

& Miles, 2006). In these studies some of the cues children use to differentiate between play and not play activities have been manipulated under experimental conditions to create playful (on the floor, adult proximal, choice) and formal (at a table, adult present, lack of choice) practice conditions. Children have been allocated to one of the practice conditions and then been involved in a familiar problem-solving task in a four-stage procedure: pre-test, practice, post-test and delayed post-test.

Results from these studies show that children in the playful practice condition perform and behave differently from children in the formal practice condition. They exhibit a significantly improved performance in time taken to complete the task. They show greater involvement in the activity as measured by the Leuven Involvement Scale (Laevers, Vandenbussche, Kog & Depondt, 1994). They exhibit greater motivation as shown by behaviours such as leaning towards the puzzle, smiling and greater focus on the activity. They also employ more purposeful problem-solving using less repetitive behaviours and try out new ways to solve problems. In addition, when children are asked to rate the practice condition they experienced they are alert to the cues being manipulated, with children in the playful practice condition rating it as far more play-like than those children in the formal practice condition.

More recent research has also demonstrated the value of this approach in evidencing children's overall wellbeing (Howard & McInnes, 2012). In this study 129 children, aged between 3 and 5 years of age, were allocated to either a 'like-play' condition or a 'not like-play' condition based on the cues described above. Children's emotional wellbeing was measured using the Leuven Involvement Scale (Laevers *et al.*, 1994), as this has been acknowledged as a measure of emotional wellbeing in young children (Laevers, 2008). Children in the 'like-play' condition scored significantly higher for emotional wellbeing than children in the 'not like-play condition'. In addition, observational data showed greater behavioural indicators for emotional wellbeing for these children.

Therefore, it would appear that if practitioners can elicit children's perceptions of play and not play activities, which are context-specific, then they can understand what is play in children's eyes. Practitioners can then work with children's perceptions of play to enable them to be more playful during activities, creating conditions that enable children to take a more playful attitude and approach to activities and facilitating a sense of wellbeing in children while undertaking activities.

The immediate and longer-term benefits of play in the context of playfulness

In previous chapters mention has been made of different theories in relation to the benefits of play. The work of Bruner (1972, 1974) highlights the importance of behavioural flexibility. He theorises that during play adverse consequences of behaviour are minimised and learning is less risky. This allows the child to try out new and increased combinations of behaviour and thinking. Likewise, Sutton-Smith argues that during play children engage in more flexible and adaptive thinking (Sutton-Smith, 1979). He subsequently presents a model of play, which states that play provides adaptive variability, which ultimately is essential for survival of the species (Sutton-Smith, 1997). These ideas are supported by research on animals, which shows that rats who are reared in playful environments display increased neural connectivity (Fagan, 1984).

More recent theoretical musings have built on this original work by Bruner and Sutton-Smith. Brown (2003) discusses the idea of compound flexibility. He theorises that the flexibility provided by play opens up opportunities for experimentation and control by the child, which increases the range of positive experiences available to the child. This increases children's sense of wellbeing, especially in relation to self-confidence, self-awareness and self-acceptance, and their flexibility in terms of thinking and problem-solving. This argument is elaborated further in the threshold and fluency theory of play proposed by Howard (2010a). In this model it is proposed that when children are feeling playful, behavioural thresholds are lowered (i.e. the level of confidence needed in a behaviour before it is enacted). This consequently results in children showing greater behavioural fluency and trying out different ways of behaving and thinking (see Figure 3.1).

However, for these theories to work in practice it necessitates children feeling playful, and, as we have argued in this chapter, this can only be achieved by understanding play from children's perspectives. If the cues children use to differentiate play from non-play activities are understood and used, then children can feel and behave playfully. In the research evidence discussed above, whereby children's cues have been manipulated to create playful and non-playful practice situations, children have consistently shown improved performance in the playful situation, and said it felt like play. Furthermore, evidence for the ideas proposed by Brown and Howard and Miles has been shown by children engaging in more purposeful behaviours during the playful practice situation and persevering with incorrect problem-solving strategies in the non-playful practice situation (McInnes *et al.*, 2009).

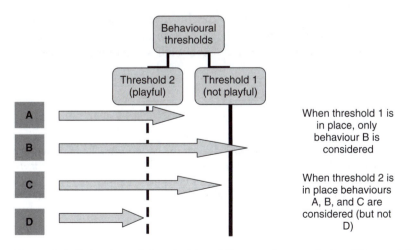

Figure 3.1 Behavioural threshold and fluency theory of play (Howard & Miles, 2008)

Conclusion

This chapter has discussed the difficulties inherent in defining play. It also highlights how traditional definitions of play are focused on the act of play as observed by adults. It is suggested that the key ingredient in children's play is the internal, affective qualities that play invokes, namely playfulness; that this affects children's attitude and approach to an activity; and that this cannot be understood by adult definitions of the observable act of play. Therefore, it is suggested that practitioners should take time to understand children's perceptions of play, which is based on cues that are context-specific. Working in this way is in keeping with current views of children and childhood, and enables practitioners to gain insight not only into the act of play but into what makes children feel playful. Furthermore, practitioners can utilise children's cues and so enable them to take a playful attitude and approach to activities.

Now that you have read the chapter

- Although differentiating between play and playfulness appears a simplistic concept, in our experience practitioners find this a difficult concept to grasp. Try explaining the distinction between play and playfulness to a colleague. This will enable you to check your understanding and develop further insight into the concepts.
- How do you think the children you work with define play, and why might this be?
- Now you need to assess whether your thoughts about their perceptions of play are accurate. Try the following activities:
  - Talk to the children about different activities in your setting. Ask them which they think are play and why. Also, remember to ask them about what they think is not play.
  - Take photographs of different activities in your setting and ask the children to sort them into whether they represent play or not play. Then talk to the children about their choices and see if any patterns emerge.

Useful further reading

Howard, J. (2010a). Making the most of children's play in the early years: The importance of children's perceptions. In P. Broadhead, J. Howard & E. Wood (Eds), *Play and Learning in the Early Years* (London: Sage Publishing Ltd., pp. 145–160).
This chapter describes the AASP in more detail. It also explains how practitioners can use this procedure in their practice.

4

The role of adults in children's play

Aims of the chapter

- To identify the important characteristics of the adult role in children's play.
- To discuss children's perceptions of the adult role in their play.
- To identify how different play practitioners engage in children's play.
- To introduce a cycle of play that may guide adults in their play interactions with children.
- To guide practitioners through a four stage reflective process on play practice.

Introduction

From the beginning of their lives children need positive relationships with their parents and carers based on sensitive and meaningful interactions. They need adults who can tune in to them, read their emotional cues and respond appropriately to them. This provides children with a secure base from which they can grow and develop (David, Goouch, Powell & Abbott, 2003; Gopnik, Meltzoff & Kuhl, 1999). Children also need this in their play (Goouch, 2010). Regardless of play practice, the role of the adult is vital. Play practitioners need to provide children with a secure base, positive regard, consistency, sensitive and meaningful interactions, and linguistic exchanges that are open and place control with the child.

This chapter will explore the important characteristics of the adult role in children's play, and identify how adults need to engage with children in their play to ensure that children have the opportunity to maximise their developmental potential. This chapter will also discuss research that has explored how children perceive adults in their play dependent upon how they engage in children's play.

Each of the play practices – educational, therapeutic and recreational – has a slightly different view of the role of the adult in children's play, and this has implications for practice. Potentially it means that there is a lack of common ground for shared practice among different play practitioners, which is especially confusing for those practitioners who cross practice boundaries either through training or in their day-to-day working lives. This chapter will discuss the underpinning principles that influence the different play practices and what this means for the practitioners. It will introduce a cycle of play that will enable practitioners to become play partners in children's play. Finally, a four-stage reflective process will be described that crosses practice boundaries and provides a basis for shared understanding of the adult role in play. This cycle of practice places the voice of the child at the centre of practice, utilising their perceptions of play in order to maximise playfulness, previously identified as the key ingredient in children's play.

Positive relationships

In order to develop and thrive children need to experience positive relationships based on sincerity, trust and respect (Whitebread, 2012). Respect for children comes from a genuine and sincere, interest and like for children, and adults who play with children need to show this acceptance of children (Landreth, 2012).

Children need people around them who treat them consistently and with positive regard, thereby laying the foundations for a good childhood and the values that will last them throughout life (Layard & Dunn, 2009). Positive relationships begin in the home with parents playing with their children (Pellegrini, 2009), and are important for the development of attachments that enable the young child to feel secure and explore the world. These positive relationships, developed through play, form the basis for future peer interactions and relationships. (See Scenario A.).

Scenario A

Colin and 8-month-old Sophie are playing with some shakers, picking them up, rattling them and giggling. Sophie throws a shaker onto the hard marble floor and laughs. She then points for Colin to get it. He picks it up and hands it back to her. She then throws it again, giggling as it bounces across the floor. Colin laughs with her and retrieves it, saying 'that was good, try a different one'. She then throws a different shaker and it makes a different sound as it bounces. The game continues as Sophie throws different shakers and waits expectantly for Colin to retrieve them one at a time. She understands the rules of the game, taking her time to throw each shaker, knowing it will be given back to her.

Communication

Adults need to be able to communicate with children both verbally and nonverbally. During play adults need to tune in to nonverbal cues in order to understand what children are thinking and feeling. For some children it may be impossible to communicate these thoughts and feelings verbally. As Landreth (2012) states, adults need to 'hear non-verbal expressions' (p. 188) to engage in meaningful communication.

In terms of verbal communication adults need to engage in meaningful dialogue that makes sense to the child. This goes beyond using vocabulary that the child understands and refers to consideration of the context in which dialogue is taking place so that children can make sense of the communication in terms of time and space. Dialogue that occurs between adults and children needs to place control of the communication with the child. Current research indicates that the type of questioning and who initiates language all reflect control within a communication frame (McInnes, Howard, Crowley & Miles, in press). In dialogue that consists primarily of closed rather than open questions, and where adults initiate conversations, control resides with the adult, and children are less likely to feel playful and to see adults as play partners. Children need to be asked open questions and feel that they can initiate language and ask questions in order to feel playful and engage adults in their play. This type of language also encourages problem-solving and exploration, important components of play.

Communication during play therefore relies on understanding and reading play cues (Else, 2009). Play cues are both nonverbal and verbal. Nonverbal cues are communicated via actions, through touch and through expressions. Verbal cues include the type of questions asked, who initiates language and the type of language used. Adults need to read the play cues given by children and be aware of the play cues they express in order to engage in play with children in a meaningful way. (See Scenario B.)

Scenario B

Child at the creative table printing with vegetables:

Child:	Can I do one?
Teacher:	Yes of course you can.
Child:	Blue and red make . . .?
Teacher:	Have a look. Make a little mark on a clean bit . . .
Child:	Purple, I've made purple! Look, it's little dots.
Teacher:	Why's it come out like that?
Child:	'Cos when you grow it the seeds just go everywhere and grow little seeds. Then the seeds have splatted all over the paper with the paint.
Teacher:	Okay!
Child:	I think it grows really high up to there and then really high up to there (pointing with finger).

Teacher:	You could be right. How could we find out?
Child:	I think we might need to do some measuring. Maybe get a ladder and climb up to measure it.
Teacher:	Hmmm.
Child:	We will do that some time. Now, what happens if I put this in here? (gesticulating with vegetable and paint)
Teacher:	I'm not sure – try it.

Dialogue between child and teacher consists of the child being in control of the dialogue and the direction and content of conversation and the teacher asking open questions to encourage exploration and problem-solving.

Time and space

Adults need to create a play space for children. This needs to be a space that is well-resourced and can accommodate children's needs and desires. It needs to have a variety of equipment and materials that can inspire children in their play (Whitebread, 2012). It needs to be a space where there are opportunities for different types of play to occur. It also needs to be a play space where children feel in control, they can express their choices and feel a sense of freedom. Some play spaces may enable children to have complete control, choice and freedom whereas other play spaces may be more constrained. However, research has demonstrated that enabling children some feeling of control, choice and freedom will still enable them to feel playful and approach activities in a play-like manner (McInnes, Howard, Miles & Crowley, 2009).

Time is a precious commodity but one that children need in order to engage in play (Williams & McInnes, 2005). Adults need to give children time to ensure that children can play at length without interruption, to lose themselves in their play. Children need time to develop a rhythm and pace to their play, which will enable them to gain depth, as well as breadth, to their play. Children also need time to communicate meaningfully during play, both with adults and their peers, and to develop relationships that enable them to feel secure and explore the world further. (See Scenario C.)

Scenario C

Will follows Marie into the playroom. There is a sand tray on the floor and beside it a small water tray. There are shelves with art materials and small world figures. There is a wooden fort in one corner of the room and a pop-up play house with dolls, puppets and role play materials. Will slowly wanders around the room looking at everything. Gradually he moves closer to the shelves and carefully picks up a toy car. He puts it down. Then he picks up another and examines it. He proceeds to do this with a variety of small world objects. He looks questioningly at Marie. She says 'whilst you are in the playroom you may choose what to play with and where'. Having been given the time to explore and the choice to do what he would like, Will then begins to take different small world objects to the sand tray. When he feels he has everything he needs he starts to play.

Playfulness

The previous chapter discussed the trait and state of playfulness in children; this can also be discussed in relation to adults. Children need playful adults to engage with them in meaningful play. Playful people are considered to make situations more stimulating, enjoyable and entertaining (Barnett, 2007). As with children, it is thought that playfulness in adults is an internal disposition that impacts on attitude and approach to an activity (Guitard, Ferland & Dutil, 2005). One assessment scale of adult playfulness, the Older Adult Playfulness scale (Yarnal & Qian, 2011) combines measurement of the trait and state of playfulness. It may be useful to consider utilising such a measure of playfulness with play practitioners. Certainly there have been calls for this within the therapeutic play field (Schaefer & Greenberg, 1997), and preliminary research within the educational play practice field has found a relationship between playfulness and ability to tolerate ambiguity within the classroom, an important prerequisite for facilitating playful encounters there (Tegano, 1990). (See Scenario D.)

Scenario D

A playful teacher is describing an available activity:

Right, listen. Outside we've got the mud. In the mud today there are some people and a carrot. You might say 'Miss B are you going mad? Why have you put people and a carrot in the mud?' Because I thought, you know the story about the enormous turnip? I thought we could change the story and have the enormous carrot! So you can act the story out with the characters and the carrot or make up your own story. Let me tell you me and Mrs C had a practice this morning and it was such fun. So have a think.

Beliefs about play

Arguably, this is the most important aspect in terms of practitioner characteristics for facilitating play and should be taken for granted. Of course, all play practitioners believe in the power of play, but at times there may be difficulties translating belief into practice. This certainly seems to be the case within educational play practice. Educational play practitioners believe in play and that children learn and develop through play, but there is evidence to suggest that practitioners' theoretical understanding of play and their role within it is not clearly understood, resulting in a mismatch between what they believe and what they do (Bennett, Wood & Rogers, 1997; Howard, 2010b). This lack of clarity is unhelpful for both practitioners and children. More recent research has shown that when practitioners are unsure about play they are less likely to join in children's play and interact with them in a playful manner, resulting in children not viewing practitioners as play partners (McInnes, Howard, Miles & Crowley, 2011). (See Scenario E.)

Scenario E

An interview with a playworker who is secure in her belief about play:

Question: How would you define play?
Answer: I would say that play is something that children do and it should be about themselves, what they want to do, not what an adult has dictated to them what playing is. That's pretty much what the playwork principles define them as, as well you know: intrinsically motivated, personally directed and freely chosen, which is probably the easiest way of defining it because they are like the playworker's Bible.
Question: What would you say your role is in children's play?
Answer: Well, going back to the playwork principles again, my role is to support and facilitate play, to observe it, to make sure children are not put in danger.

White, 2012

Children's perceptions of the adult role in play

As discussed in the previous chapter, by using multiple methodologies it has been shown that children use cues to differentiate between activities they see as play and those they see as not play. One of the cues they use is adult presence. Previous research has shown that children tend to define activities as play when an adult is not present and not play when an adult is present (Howard, 2002). They also define an activity as not play if there is adult evaluation of the play process or product of the play process. Research discussed in the previous chapter has shown how manipulating the cues children use, including adult presence, to differentiate between play and not play activities to create playful and formal practice conditions results in differences in children's performance and behaviour during a problem-solving task (McInnes *et al.*, 2009).

Further research focused on the cue of adult presence has looked at this phenomenon in more detail (McInnes, Howard, Miles & Crowley, 2010). This study manipulated the cues children use to define play and not play to create four practice conditions: playful (adult proximal, on floor, choice); formal (adult present, at table, no choice); playful with adult present (adult present, on floor, choice); and formal with adult proximal (adult proximal, at table, no choice). Again a familiar problem-solving task was employed across a pre-test, practice, post-test, delayed post-test procedure. The results showed that in the two practice conditions with the adult proximal rather than present children showed increased performance, increased involvement, more behaviours conducive to learning and more likelihood to rate the practice conditions as play. Children in the two practice conditions with the adult present did not show these improvements in performance or involvement, exhibited behaviour that did not aid learning and were less likely to rate the practice conditions as play.

Research into children's perceptions of play has shown their perceptions are dependent upon the type of setting they experience, with children in less structured and more playful settings making fewer play and not play distinctions. A further study has shown that practitioners' understanding about play and their role in children's play influences how they interact with children, which in turn influences children's perceptions of the adult role (McInnes *et al.*, 2011). In this study it was shown that when play practitioners have a secure understanding of children's play and their role within it, they interact with children in a way that affords them choice and control. This enables the children to view practitioners as play partners and to not use the cue of adult presence to differentiate between play and not play. Conversely, when play practitioners do not have a secure understanding of play and their role within it, then the adults, rather than the children, control the play. Children are then less likely to see adults as play partners and more likely to use the cue of adult presence to differentiate between play and not play.

This is further supported by a study looking at children and young people's views of playworkers (Manwaring, 2006). Recreational play practitioners have a secure understanding of play and their role within it, underpinned by a set of play principles. As a result children perceive these play practitioners as enabling them to have freedom and choice. They know they are in control of their play but they want the adults to join in. They also recognise differences between recreational play practitioners and other adults they come into contact with such as teachers, stating that they had less freedom with teachers. However, this is balanced by younger children finding it more difficult to differentiate between different types of play practitioners, presumably reflecting the differences in settings and practice they experience. These differences are a reflection of different underpinning principles and practice that impact on the role of the adult, and these will now be discussed.

Educational play practice

When teaching through play, practitioners are encouraged to engage in a pedagogy of play (Wood & Attfield, 2005). This necessitates that practitioners understand the importance of play in children's development and that they plan an appropriate play-based curriculum with appropriate play activities, which should be balanced between those that are child-initiated and those that are adult-initiated. The practitioners are encouraged to intervene when appropriate to support and extend children's learning as they play. They are also expected to observe, monitor and assess children's learning and development as they engage in play activities. Overall, the adult role is focused on utilising play as a vehicle for learning, although without explicitly stating how they should do this.

In the literature there is guidance on the different roles educational practitioners may take when engaging in educational play practice. This guidance ranges from being uninvolved to being a co-player to being a director of children's play (Johnson, Christie & Wardle, 2005; Jones & Reynolds, 1992; VanHoorn, Nourot, Scales & Alward, 2007). Sheridan, Howard and Alderson (2011) provide a list of roles that adults might adopt:

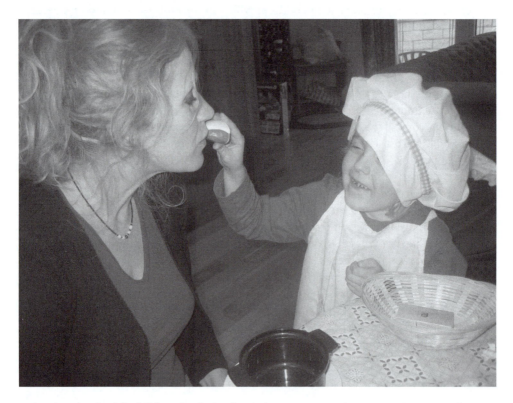

Being involved with children in their play is important, as it communicates to them how much we value their ideas

- *play partner* – becoming an equal in play;
- *observer* – observing children's development and progress;
- *admirer* – showing that you value play;
- *facilitator* – easing play along;
- *model* – showing how play materials might be used;
- *mediator* – resolving conflict;
- *safety officer* – ensuring safety (pp. 71–2).

This is potentially confusing for educational practitioners as they grapple with deciding which role to take, when to take it and how to execute it. As research conducted with educational play practitioners has shown, they often neglect the role of play partner during play interactions with children (Howard, 2010b). This has implications in relation to the cue of adult presence when defining play. As described previously, if children do not see the adult as a play partner then they will use the cue of adult presence as a defining feature of play. When they do see the adult as a play partner they do not use the cue (McInnes *et al.*, 2011).

Therapeutic play practice

Non-directive play therapy is underpinned by Axline's eight principles (Axline, 1989). These are:

- developing a warm and friendly relationship with the child;
- accepting the child as she or he is;
- establishing a feeling of permission in the relationship so that the child feels free to express her of his feelings completely;
- recognising the feelings the child is expressing and reflecting these feelings back so that the child gains insight into their behaviour;
- believing in the child's ability to solve his/her problems and allowing the child to do so;
- letting the child lead the play;
- ensuring that therapy is a gradual process;
- placing limitations to ensure that therapy is based in reality and that the child is aware of this.

These principles ensure clarity for the adult role in play (West, 1996).

Within therapeutic play practice the role of the adult is to respect the child and establish a relationship with the child. Play is free from adult direction as the child is in control and leads the play. The adult utilises play as communication, not to lead communication between adult and child but to reflect back to the child what they are communicating. Again the locus of control within the communicative exchange is with the child. In addition, the role of the adult is to provide a safe place in which the child can play and communicate and time to do so. The adult also needs to be playful and have a sense of humour so that they can share in playful experiences with the child (Landreth, 2012).

Recreational play practice

Recreational play practice also has a set of underpinning principles, which are clearly articulated. These are stated as:

- Play is a necessity and fundamental for development.
- Play is a freely chosen process and children are in control.
- Practitioners need to support and facilitate the play process.
- Practitioners act as 'advocates' for children's play.
- Practitioners support the creation of a play space.
- Practitioners need up-to-date knowledge of the play process.
- Practitioners are aware of their effect on children's play.
- Practitioners extend children's play appropriately.

Conway, 2008

Again, these principles, clearly understood by practitioners, ensure clarity for the adult role in play. Adults understand play as a freely chosen process in which the child is in control. They are aware that they do not have different roles as such, or have to choose between them, but they help create an environment in which children can play and generally do not interfere in that process other than to support the play children are engaged in. Adults are aware of how they may affect children's play, and are encouraged to be playful in their interactions with children. It is also understood that adults will keep up to date in their knowledge about play, thus enabling them to interact meaningfully and to act to stand up for the right for children to play.

Comparing play practices

As previous chapters have outlined, different play practitioners have different theoretical understandings of play. There is some shared theoretical underpinning, but generally different play practitioners view play differently. This has led to differences in ways of working. Both recreational and therapeutic play practice have developed principles that underpin their practice while educational play practice has developed a pedagogy of play. The principles underpinning recreational and therapeutic play practice have resulted in clarity in the adult role within children's play. Practitioners within recreational play practice leave play to children, they help create an environment for play and they support children's play appropriately but do not interfere in their play. Practitioners within therapeutic play practice again leave the play to children and adults communicate and reflect on the play process with children. There is less clarity concerning the adult role within educational play practice. Adults engage in multiple decision-making regarding what and how children play and their role within that. This creates confusion for adults and cues for children regarding the role of the adult in play.

Playfulness and the role of the adult in children's play

In the previous chapter the argument was made that it is the internal, affective qualities of play that are important therapeutically and for development, such as enthusiasm, motivation and willingness to engage (Moyles, 1989; Rogers & Sluss, 1999). It was also argued that to understand this it is necessary to differentiate between play, as an observable act, and playfulness, as an approach and attitude to an activity. This requires practitioners to not only observe children's play but to listen to children and understand play from their perspective. Children use cues to differentiate between play and not play, and this is dependent upon experience. Research has shown that utilising these cues affects a child's attitude and approach to an activity – their levels of playfulness. In order to maintain levels of playfulness and for children to derive the full benefits from approaching an activity playfully, it is important that adults understand their role within the play cycle.

Playfulness and the play cycle

Playing with others and deriving the benefits of play is dependent upon maintaining feelings of playfulness. To achieve this, participants in play need to recognise and maintain the flow of play through the play cycle. The idea of a play cycle with parti-cipants reading and responding to play cues comes from the work of Sturrock and Else (1998). They posited that initially a player delivers a play cue that they have choice and control over. This is issued as an invitation to play. The play partner responds to the cue. This response must be appropriate, based on the child's interest, otherwise the play will be terminated. The response to the play cue by the co-player is then delivered back to the player and the cycle of play is maintained (see Figure 4.1).

To explain this in play terms the cue given might be a simple action cue, for example, playing catch. A child might throw a ball as an invitation to play. The ball might be thrown back, in which case the cue has been received and responded to appropriately. The ball might be kicked back, again appropriate receiving and responding to the initial play cue. In both of these examples the play cycle is maintained. However, the play might be thrown to one side or dropped, terminating the play.

Another example could be through construction play. A child might be building a tower of bricks. The child might hand a brick to the adult, an invitation to join in the play. The adult might respond to the play cue by taking the brick and placing on the tower, joining in the construction and maintaining the play flow. However, the adult might take the brick, and in an attempt to turn it into a teaching moment say 'how many will this make?' To the child this might be an inappropriate response, thereby interrupting the flow of play and terminating the play cycle.

The play cycle also has resonance with Garvey's work on play episodes (Garvey, 1991). Garvey described how children seem to have a series of themes, or action sequences, that they play out with little discussion of how, what or what. These sequences have a clear flow or cycle to them, and using play cues as described above would explain the process of play episodes. Again, inappropriate responses would

Figure 4.1
The play cycle

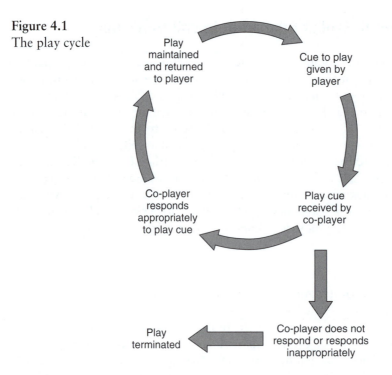

terminate play episodes. There are also links with flow states (Csikszentmihalyi, 1979, 1990), where having choice and control over activities leads to deep concentration, pleasure and satisfaction. It is often referred to as 'getting lost' in the activity, and this is often observed in children who are deeply engaged in play episodes that are within their control. This involvement and engagement in an activity can be measured using the Leuven Involvement Scale (Laevers, Vandenbussche, Kog & Depondt, 1994), as described in Chapter 7. Research has shown that when children are deeply involved in activities they view as play, which leads to deep-level learning and greater wellbeing (Howard & McInnes, 2012; McInnes *et al.*, 2009).

The role of the adult in the play cycle is a demanding one. Practitioners must constantly reflect on their reaction to a cue to ensure they maintain the cycle of play. This is embedded within therapeutic play practice whereby the play therapist is constantly aware of and reflecting on their responses to children's play (West, 1996). Practitioners constantly need to ask themselves 'what is behind my response?' 'Is this for my benefit?' as in the construction play example given above whereby a developmental outcome was clearly in evidence? Or is the response based on the child's intention for the play? It is only in this latter response that the play cycle and playfulness can be maintained and that children can deeply engage in a play activity. In this way the benefits of playfulness can be achieved.

Reflecting on play practice

Practitioners can, therefore, utilise this knowledge to inject playfulness into a variety of activities and situations and to reduce children's use of the cue of adult presence to differentiate between play and not-play activities, resulting in greater playfulness. Using the research and ideas presented in this chapter and Chapter 7, practitioners can engage in a four-stage reflective process on practice, which may be utilised by all play practitioners, thereby creating some common ground in play practice. These stages are:

- informed practice;
- utilisation of children's perceptions of play;
- reflection on children's perceptions of play;
- reflection on the adult role in play.

Informed practice

Informed practice means being aware of the characteristics of the adult role in children's play: positive relationships founded on respect and security; clear nonverbal and verbal communication where control is shared by adults and children; provision of time and space for play; a sense of playfulness in encounters with children; and an informed belief and understanding of play. These characteristics need to be understood and articulated by all practitioners. Informed practice also means understanding play from children's perspectives; that children use cues to make play and not play distinctions; and these are informed by what children experience, especially in relation to the adult role. By understanding that children use cues, and by being willing to work with them, adults can create a dialogue of practice around playfulness and enable children to take a playful attitude and approach to activities.

Utilisation of children's perceptions of play

The cues children use to define play and not play activities are clearly described in the literature. However, practitioners could confirm the cues children are using in the setting by routinely take photographs of the children in their setting. Photographs could be taken of the children playing at different activities, at different times of the day, with the adults and with their peers. Children could then be asked to reflect on the play they see in the photographs. Practitioners can then talk with children about why they have categorised the photographs the way they have. This information will enable them to identify how children perceive play activities in their setting and what cues they are using to do so. Practitioners will then be able to work with these cues to modify the provision available and their play practice.

Reflection on children's perceptions of play

Reflecting on children's perceptions of play relies on practitioners being able to stand back and take an honest appraisal of their practice; this may be difficult for practitioners. Depending on the cues being used, it may necessitate practitioners reflecting on the type of activities available for children and how they are available for children.

It may mean practitioners having to consider how much choice and control children they allow children, and also what is permissible within the setting in which they work. It will also require them to reflect on themselves as practitioners within therapeutic play practice – this is termed 'self-understanding', ultimately resulting in 'self-acceptance' (Landreth, 2012), possibly something that all play practitioners should be striving for.

Reflection on the adult role in play

Reflection on the adult role in play means reflecting on this in relation to children's perceptions of the adult role. It means reflecting on whether children see adults as play partners, and if not why not, and, even if they do, how this can be improved upon. This will be dependent upon accurately reading the play cues given by the child and responding appropriately. Adults may want to consider what kind of relationship they have with the children in their setting and how positive it is. They may wish to look at how they communicate and play with children, possibly by video or audio recording some play episodes, a common practice within therapeutic play practice. Identifying how they respond to play cues and the type of language used, questions asked and who initiates and controls interactions and play will illuminate play and communicative practice between adults and children. The time children have to play and the play space provided should also be considered, and practitioners will need to reflect on their own playfulness. Embarking on this reflective cycle of play practice and utilising a conceptual framework based on children's perceptions of play should result in practitioners questioning and developing their own beliefs and understanding about play.

Conclusion

This chapter has identified the characteristics needed by play practitioners in order to facilitate play with children. It has also identified how these characteristics impact on children's perceptions of the adult role in play, and how adults may or may not be seen as play partners by children. Discussion has focused on how different play practices have different underpinning principles that impact on the role of the adult, and how this may result in differences in the way different play practitioners might be viewed by children. Finally, a cycle of play practice has been introduced that is based on children's perceptions of play. This enables practitioners to work with children to co-construct an atmosphere and environment that reduces cue distinctions, blurs the boundaries between play and not play and enables a more playful attitude and approach to activities. This approach also blurs the boundaries between different play practices and helps play practitioners work together to maximise playfulness for children. This approach results in a shared understanding of play, one based on playfulness and not the observable act of play. It results in a shared understanding of the adult role, one that maximises playfulness rather than providing play activities.

For educational play practitioners, it frees them from considerations of *when* to intervene in play, moving the focus to *how* to intervene in play to facilitate playfulness. For therapeutic play practitioners, it builds on principles concerned with listening to the child and letting them take the lead in play, as the starting point for practice is understanding and using children's understanding of play. For recreational play practitioners, it also works with the play principles concerned with the child being in control and builds on adults supporting and facilitating play to adults supporting and facilitating playfulness.

Now that you have read the chapter

- What kinds of role do you generally adopt when engaging with children in play? What do you think are your strengths and weaknesses? Make a list and engage in some CPD to develop your practice.
- How do you think your practice might contribute to how the children you work with view play? Are there changes you could make to your practice that might alter how the children view play?
- How well do you think you can 'read' children's cues to play?
- Reflect on the strengths and weaknesses you listed above and see if any directly relate to how children might view play. Maybe you need to add to the list and make further changes?

Useful further reading

Sturrock, G. & Else, P. (1998) The playground as therapeutic space: Playwork as healing [known as the 'Colorado Paper']. In G. Sturrock and P. Else (2005) *Therapeutic Playwork: Reader One* (Sheffield: Ludemos).
Although the terminology used in this text may not be familiar, it provides an excellent and detailed account of the play drive and play cycle.

5	# The play environment

Aims of the chapter

- To consider the value of sensory, symbolic and role play experiences from a developmental perspective.
- To consider some important features of the play environment.
- To explore some of the benefits associated with particular play materials.

Introduction

In Chapter 2 we explored the nature of children's learning and development from birth to adolescence. We considered the way in which children's play changes over time and how these changes both reflect and contribute to children's development. While different theorists emphasise different areas of development or different mechanisms for learning, a pattern of development in play is apparent in these accounts. This pattern is usefully captured in the Embodiment, Projection and Role (EPR) developmental paradigm proposed by Jennings (1999), who suggests that we all pass through these play stages and that each type of play experience is vital in offering intrinsic learning opportunities.

Embodiment Stage – Here the child's early experiences are largely physical and are understood and expressed through the senses. The child is developing their bodily self, learning to differentiate and organise perceptual experiences. This stage is important to a developing sense of identity and much involves experiences between the child and primary caregiver.

- Activities here might include: fine and gross motor movement, music and singing, experiencing different sounds and textures.
- Theorists: Attachment (Bowlby), Sensorimotor stage and practice play (Piaget), oral stage (Freud), autocosmic play (Erikson) and enactive representation (Bruner).

Projective Stage – Here the child begins to relate to the world outside of the self through engaging with toys and objects within their environment. They learn about the properties of objects and develop the ability to use materials symbolically in their play. Understanding the impact of their actions on the world around them is important in the development of independence, confidence and self-esteem. Children gradually begin to understand the perspectives of others.

- Activities here might include: working with sand, water, paints or crayons, small world materials like cars and people, block play.
- Theorists: Early symbolic play (Piaget), microspheric and macrospheric play (Erikson) and iconic representation (Bruner).

Role Stage – Here the child takes on roles rather than projecting them through toys and objects. Children may model behaviour, trying on and trying out ideas and actions with the safety of the unreal world. Enacting experiences can bring us closer to understanding real-life experience. This type of play allows us to learn about our self identify and our social identity. It allows us to understand the nuances and complexities of human behaviour in the real world through drama and play.

- Activities here might include: dressing up, role play games, making masks of characters or emotions, dramatising stories.
- Theorists: Symbolic play (Piaget), macrospheric play (Erikson) and symbolic representation (Bruner).

Jennings proposes that progression through these stages is generally sequential and complete by the age of 7, but that we return to each stage throughout childhood as our identities continue to develop.

Key to the paradigm is that each type of play is vital to the initial and continued development of a healthy sense of self and emotional wellbeing. Emotional wellbeing underpins development across domains, and play is a key way to support this. Difference and diversity can prevent, disrupt or slow progression through embodied, projective and role play types. Youell (2009) describes how the play of children who have experienced abuse, deprivation or neglect is often severely inhibited, and urges

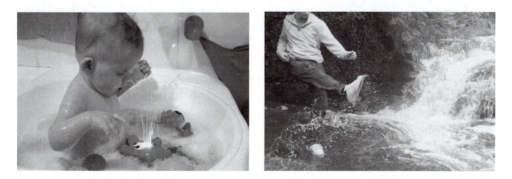

The sensory experience of water is a source of fascination from infancy through to adolescence

practitioners to consider both the behavioural and affective elements of play. She highlights how the play of these children 'can look like play whilst being devoid of any creativity, symbolic meaning or sense of playfulness' (Youell, 2009, p. 190). Observing and assessing children's play in some of the ways described in Chapter 7 can be useful here in order ensure the provision that provides opportunities for success and challenge.

Features of the play environment

As we saw in Chapter 3, procedural elements of the environment and the way in which we interact with children are both highly influential in determining whether or not an activity is seen as play or not play. This, in turn, influences children's experience of the here and now (the 'being' element of play) and any developmental potential of this experience in the longer term (the 'becoming' element of play). The physical environment we provide for the children in our care, however, is also important, as are the materials contained within this.

It goes without saying that, first and foremost, the environment and materials must be considered safe for the children with whom we work. This will necessarily involve initial and ongoing professional evaluation based on our knowledge of each child, as well as reflection on previous experiences we have had in our settings. Challenge and risk are both important features of play, however, and we must be careful not to restrict the opportunities we provide by being overly cautious. Tovey (2007) usefully distinguishes between environments that are 'safe as possible' and environments that are 'safe enough', highlighting that, often, ensuring that children are completely free from risk leads to under-stimulation, feelings of incompetence and, crucially, limited opportunities to develop and manage key risk-taking skills. Tovey proposes that a safe environment is one where safety is not seen as protecting children from all possible harm but rather one where children are safe to explore.

Children enjoy playing in a variety of different spaces and places, and while to a certain extent these might be shaped by what is available in our professional contexts, key to our provision is that we consider what the space available affords children to do (Kytta, 2004). A room packed with equipment might look attractive and well resourced but may not leave scope for any real 'playing' to take place. While it might be necessary to have certain fixed materials (for example, painting materials near to the sink or where there is an easy clean floor), it can be best to avoid making unnecessary boundaries so as to enable as much independent choice and control as is possible. Broadhead (2010) describes the importance of early years classrooms having an 'anything you want it to be space', where children are in direct control over the theme and content of their play. Through her research, she demonstrates that this leads to more sophisticated social interaction and richer play content. Jennings (1999) similarly argues that play spaces should include a magical and symbolic space where things can are allowed and children are safe to express themselves.

Both of these propositions remind us that essential to our professional play practice is that children are able to form and transform at will (Drummond, 1999). Children value the opportunity to choose whether to play in larger open spaces or small enclosed ones, and many activities can occur in or outdoors. Early years curricula across the UK and beyond emphasise the value of outdoor play, and most recreational playwork is provided outdoors. However, the benefits of outdoor play can be extended beyond this to children in hospital or even, where a suitable space is available and confidentiality permits, to children receiving therapy or counselling. Outdoor play and the natural environment are discussed further later on in this chapter.

In terms of materials, again, facilitating choice and control is important. Some early years settings, such as Steiner-Waldorf, have a preference toward natural over man-made materials, and here it would be unusual to find dolls or wheeled toys as children would be expected to construct what they needed for their play themselves or to use materials symbolically.

Natural materials are also used in many of the activities children can choose in a Montessori setting. In recent years traditional toys made from wood have regained popularity, and while these can often be sturdier than their plastic counterparts their play value is relatively constant. Treasure baskets filled with natural materials, as suggested by Goldschmied and Jackson (1994), invite sensory exploration, but children are equally propelled to explore man-made objects that might be included, like stickle-bricks or a wheeled toy. Toys or materials can be open-ended and have multiple uses, like blocks, cardboard boxes and junk materials or fabric scraps. These 'loose parts'

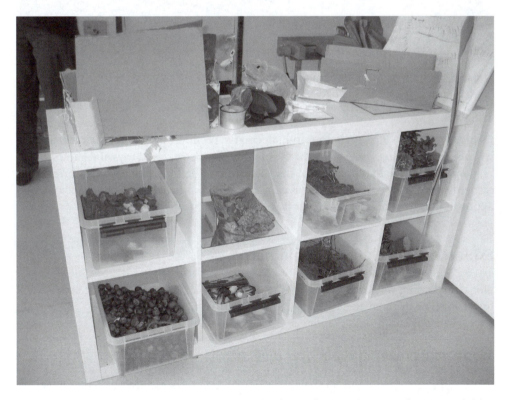

In this Reggio Emilia classroom, attractive displays of natural materials are available for children to use on a daily basis for art, craft and creative play

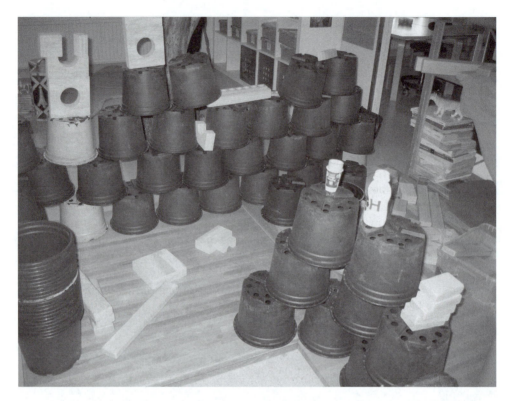

Loose parts such as these basic plant pots can provide a range of creative play opportunities

(Nicholson, 1971) allow children to play creatively in as many different ways as they wish. Some children, however, might thoroughly enjoy structured toys and games where outcomes are predictable or where instructions can be followed. Toys and materials certainly need not be expensive or commercially produced, and children will find opportunities to play with whatever is to hand.

Exploring the value of certain play types

Notwithstanding the immediate benefits of feeling playful, the following section will focus on some of the benefits associated with certain play types.

Music, movement and physical play

The benefits of music for children's development are well documented. Hallam (2010) reviews the potential for music to impact on children's development across domains, and evaluates rigorous evidence linking music to language development, literacy and numeracy skills, measures of general intelligence and attainment, creativity as well as motivation and self-esteem. Evidence collected in medical settings has demonstrated how music serves as a means of distraction and relaxation, and children who are able to play music prior to and after their surgery report less pain and stress and recover more quickly (Young *et al.*, 2010).

Music and movement are naturally paired, and Goddard-Blythe (2004) proposes that they contribute to proprioceptive learning – knowledge about the physical self in action. Experiencing music and movement facilitates progression from reflex action through to controlled, balanced and co-ordinated movement.

Children learn about their relative size through physical play, and we can observe their growing bodily awareness as they attempt to climb in and out of boxes, baskets or wheeled toys. Understanding other physical capacities such as balance and co-ordination continues throughout childhood. Unusual reflex patterns or immature vestibular functioning is often a feature of children with developmental disorders such as dyslexia and dyspraxia, ADHD (or other attention/behaviour problems), anxiety and depression. Children with concentration- or motor-related problems who participated in a music and movement programme entitled 'return to balance' demonstrated notable improvements in physical and psychological development (Niklasson *et al.*, 2010). Early musical activities involve children interacting with their primary caregiver and then peers and other adults. These activities promote the development of key social skills as well as making them feel good about themselves.

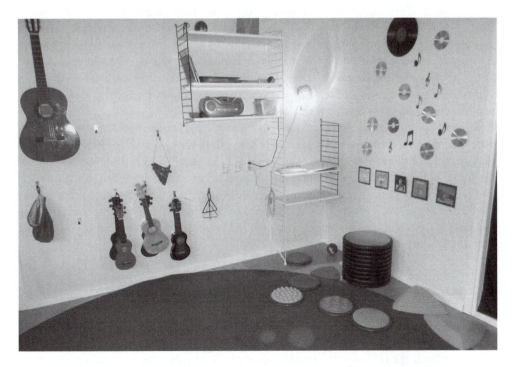

This attractive space invites children to experience music and movement. The positioning of materials at appropriate heights means choice and control are maximised

Sand, water and other sensory play activities

In much the same way as music and movement, sensory play activities enable children to learn about their physical self and the way in which they are able to impact on the world around them. From birth, babies use their sense of smell to identify their primary caregiver, and throughout these early months they delight in different sights, sounds and tactile experiences. As was previously noted, in the EPR model (Jennings, 1999), sensory play activity is an important precursor to other types of play. The world is full of sensory information, and while it was previously felt that this may lead to infants experiencing a big 'blooming, buzzing confusion' (James, 1890), research has demonstrated that even very young babies are very good at organising this information. The type of environment children experience plays a key role in the development of a healthy and balanced sense of self.

During heuristic play, Goldschmied and Jackson (1994) propose that infants learn about themselves and their environment via the exploration of sensory materials, which, to avoid the 'buzzing confusion' should be kept simplistic and be self-selected. This enables the child to control the level and pace at which they receive sensory stimulation. Children with sensory dysfunction often exhibit unusual play patterns, lower levels of playfulness (Bundy *et al.*, 2007) and often play in repetitive ways (Dunn, 1997).

Shaaf and Miller (2005) propose that sensory–motor development is an important precursor to learning; that the child's interaction with the environment shapes the development of the brain and nervous system; and that meaningful sensory–motor activity plays a significant role in brain plasticity. They go on to describe effective features of the sensory integration approach, which includes providing a playful environment with opportunities for challenge and success, where the child is in control of the activity and the therapist takes the child's lead, picking up on behavioural cues and suggestions. Here again, we can see how these principles mirror those of effective play practice across professional contexts.

Sensory activities might include play with water, clay, sand, objects and materials of different textures or items with a distinctive smell. It is important to distinguish sand play from sand therapy at this juncture, however. Lowenfeld (1979) developed one of the most widely adopted sand therapy techniques, known as the World Technique. It involves children choosing miniature objectives to create sand tray scenes that reflect their attempts to work through issues that are witnessed by the therapist. Sand therapy is a particular technique for which experienced counsellors and therapists undertake additional comprehensive training.

Art, drawing and creative play

Children enjoy mark-making from a very early age and, often, their first attempts involve the smearing of food over a highchair surface or table top. They appear to delight in both the texture they experience and the growing understanding that their actions are causing the patterns and marks to appear. Vygostky (1978) proposes that early marks are indicative of children's first attempts at symbolic communication.

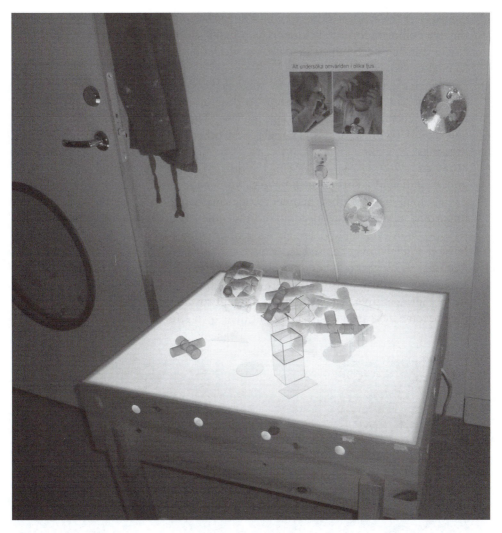

The use of light and mirrored materials can provide a range of interesting sensory experiences. In this picture, also note the well-considered porthole window in the lower section of the door. This allowed children to create a more private play space while at the same time enabled discreet adult monitoring

Schirrmacher (2002) proposes that children's mark-making follows a developmental pattern from various levels of scribbling at age 1–3 years, pre-schematic drawings at age 4–6 years, schematic drawings at age 7–9 years and an emphasis on realistic drawing at 9–11 years. A description of each level is provided below:

- *Scribbling* (1–3 years) – initially, scribbles are largely dots and lines, and enjoyment is mainly about being able to make a mark on the page. Gradually more control is gained over the mark-making tool and intent becomes apparent. Circles are often the first complete form to be drawn. Gradually scribbles may become named, and circles and lines are joined to represent the human form in tadpole-like figures (cephalopods).

- *Pre-schematic* (4–6 years) – at this stage depiction of the human form becomes more complex. Children may begin to develop an individual style of drawing, building schema for use in drawings later on. They may begin to combine shapes and figures to draw scenes. Triangles and other shapes become integrated into drawings.
- *Schematic* (7–9 years) – drawings reflect a child's conceptual or schematic understanding of a particular thing (e.g. women are depicted as wearing dresses or having long hair). Other people recognising what has been drawn becomes important, and drawings become more detailed and decorative. A personalised style becomes evident, and similar ways of drawing particular things (e.g. people, houses, animals) may be used repetitively.
- *Realism* (9–12 years) – children show concern for detail and perspective, and struggle to produce pictures that are realistic rather than conceptually or intellectually representative. Their drawings attempt to show action and movement, and they become increasingly critical about their own efforts.

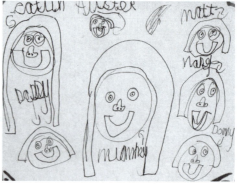

Here you can clearly see the progress in this child's human figure drawing from his early tadpoles or 'cephalopods' at aged 4 to a more personal schematic style at aged 6

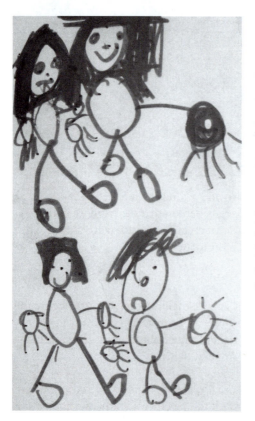

Drawing offers many opportunities for the development of fine motor control, and is also an important precursor to development in other areas such as literacy and numeracy (Worthington, 2007). Children who are offered playful opportunities to draw, draw more often, for more sustained periods of time and demonstrate more highly developed mark-making skills (Ring, 2010).

Some scholars argue that the content of children's drawings can be indicative of children's understanding of the world around them or their emotional state (e.g. Skybo, Wenger & Su, 2007). However, research has demonstrated that drawing is generally symbolic (for example, children make more elaborate block models of the human body than they initially draw). The dangers of interpretation are highlighted in Chapter 7.

As children begin to develop symbolic ability, they begin to enjoy other creative activities such as clay or junk modelling and block building. Here, given the opportunity to make choices and direct their own activities, they are able to develop their imaginative skills and creativity.

Of importance to professional practice is that we pay attention to process over product, and any outcome and judgement of this outcome must be left to the child. Materials such as Lego blocks are of particular value as they can be built following pictorial or written instructions or used in an open-ended way. Construction and creative play also has socio-emotional benefits, and Whitebread, Basilio, Kuvalja and Verma (2012) report a Lego therapy programme that led to reduced maladaptive behaviour among children with autistic spectrum disorders.

Role play and pretence

Children's initial pretend play generally involves using small world toys such as cars, dolls house sets, garages or farms with small animals. Here children demonstrate projective play, where they are playing with objects outside of the self. They demonstrate an ability to see themselves as separate from the world, but are not yet fully able to allow one thing to stand for another, the play items being used to mirror their 'real' use (Sheridan, Howard & Alderson, 2010). Jennings (1999) considers miniature toys to be of particular value, enabling children to safely deal with overwhelming experiences, the size of the toy making things seem more manageable. Small toys are also beneficial in offering opportunities for pretence at the hospital bedside.

Gradually, as symbolic ability grows, children can make equipment for their play using a variety of materials in novel ways. For example, early years educators may earnestly endeavour to disallow guns in their environments, but if required children can often be observed making these from sticks, blocks or their fingers. Allowing one thing to stand for something else is associated with a move away from geocentrism and the ability to understand another person's perspective or to show theory of mind (Whitebread, 2012).

Role play begins to emerge at around 3 to 4 years and, like projective activities, often involves playing out known activities like mums and dads or shops. Here children take on familiar roles and demonstrate their understanding of what this role means to them. This then progresses into more imaginative role play or dramatic play, where children may develop complex scripts and stories involving a wide range of characters, both real and imaginary. A variety of fabrics, scarves, hats and other inexpensive everyday materials can be used effectively as props.

The benefits of socio-dramatic play are well documented. Children develop key social skills, the semantic and pragmatic elements of language and can try on and try out a variety of emotions. In particular, socio-dramatic play experiences offer invaluable opportunities for the development of self-regulatory behaviours, particularly for children with attention or behavioural issues (Elias & Berk, 2002). Even older children may continue to enjoy dressing up or trying on new identities, and may express this by playing with their own self-image, through playful interactions with peers or more formally through drama or theatre.

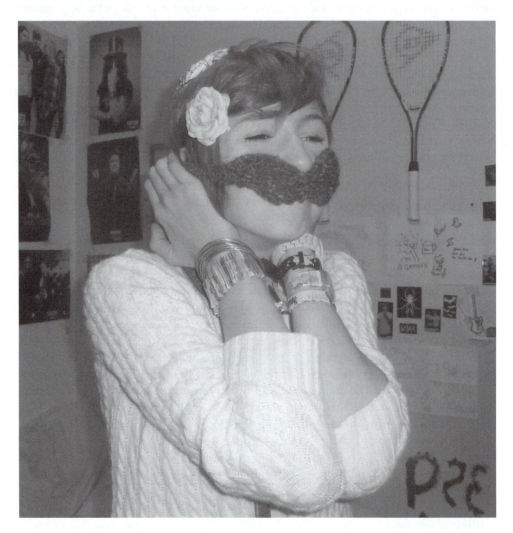

This teenager had great fun knitting herself woolly moustaches! In the background, also note the personalisation of the bedroom walls

We may not always feel comfortable, however, with the themes or actions contained in children's socio-dramatic play, and Wood (2010) highlights that in providing play experiences that offer freedom and autonomy, we must be prepared for the dark side of play, associated with the subversion of social rules and norms.

As was highlighted in Chapter 2, puppets are a valuable play resource across professional contexts. They can often bridge the gap between projective and role activity and, in addition, they provide wonderful sensory experiences as they are often made from soft fur fabric or a variety of other materials that afford tactile exploration. Children can talk through a puppet, allowing distance from the message being communicated, and the value of puppets in therapeutic work and preparation for surgery in medical contexts is well documented (Schaefer, 2011). Puppets can also be used to tell or create therapeutic stories (Sunderland, 2001) or as a means of reaching out to children when talking about their feelings (Howard & Elton, 2009).

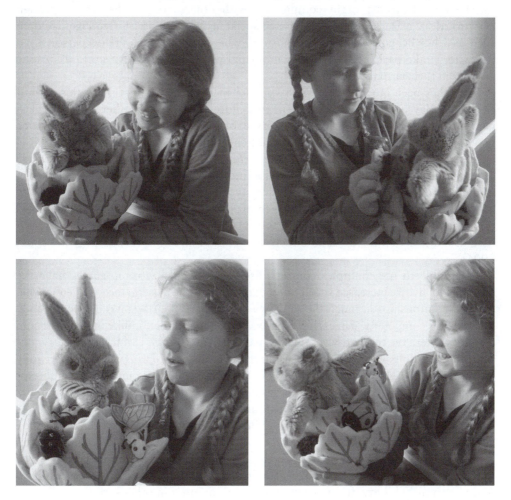

Puppets are an excellent resource and offer opportunities for sensory, projective and role play

Children enjoy being told stories but also benefit from making up their own stories. A variety of techniques can be employed to facilitate this, for example, by starting a narrative and using 'I wonder what happens next . . .?' Fernyhough (2008, in Cowie, 2012) proposes that stories are like time travel, allowing children to understand the past, the future and to imagine all kinds of possibilities. This can be particularly useful for children who appear to have lost hope that situations can change.

ICT and virtual play

Over recent years there has been a remarkable rise in the amount of electronic gaming devices available on the market as well as the incorporation of gaming applications on mobile phones and tablet computers. Computer games have now extended to those that can be played against or in conjunction with others around the world through networked sites. There are also play-based social networking sites for younger children such as Club Penguin or Moshi Monsters, where children can create personalised characters, take part in games and win virtual prizes but also visit and talk to one another in their virtual worlds.

There has been much debate as to whether increased participation in this type of electronic play occurs at the detriment to children engaging in other forms of play, particularly physical outdoor play. One issue, of course, is that much electronic game play can be sedentary and can prevent children from getting enough physical exercise, influencing body mass and weight (Epstein et al., 2007). Newer gaming devices have attempted to incorporate physical exercise into the gaming experience, for example, using technology with motion sensors. This type of device has been used successfully in studies of physical rehabilitation, which maximise on children's motivation toward this type of activity (Deutsch et al., 2008). Handheld gaming devices have also been used as a distraction for children undergoing painful medical procedures (Patel et al., 2006).

Being able to use multiple handsets also means that electronic games have the potential to involve increased social interaction, and can be a useful means of enhancing familial relationships in much the same way as perhaps board games. A recent study of children's computer use in early years classrooms found that, unlike other classroom activities where the teacher was often seen as a barrier to play, children were far more accepting of adults while they were using the computer, accepting them more readily as play partners (Howard, Miles & Rees-Davies, 2012). There may be a number of reasons for this: the computer may act as a mediator for control over the activity, or children may simply feel more confident and competent in this type of activity, thus balancing what is the often biased adult–child power relationship. Children often enjoy explaining to adults how to use particular computer programs, and this can be a useful means of opening a conversation or developing relationships with them.

A further criticism of increased use of electronic games has been that their solitary nature prevents children from engaging with one another in other types of play, thus reducing the opportunities they have for developing key social skills. Jarvis (2009) makes a very powerful case for this in relation to decreased engagement in rough and

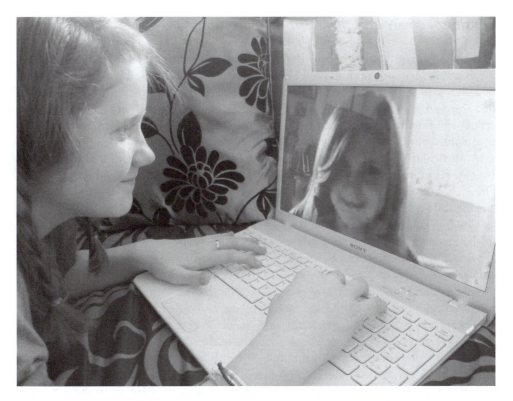

Talking to friends online has become a regular form of communication for young people

tumble play, arguing that increased anti-social behaviour in society may reflect this trend. However, with the increased level of networked games and the ability to communicate both directly via a headset or via text messaging during game play can provide children who might otherwise not interact with peers a safe space to try out their developing social skills.

Of course, the 'safety' of being behind a screen (computer, mobile phone or tablet) can mean that children fail to consider the impact that their messages might have on others or feel that this is something other than 'real' interaction. The dangers of this are very real, and cyberbullying has sadly become an increasing problem, causing distress to many children and young people (Cowie, 2012). The potential scope of cyberbullying extends from negative social network messages, emails and texts, as well as exclusion from groups via the same means. Whereas traditional bullying may take place on the way to school, on the way home or during breaks, cyberbullying could occur throughout the whole of a child's day. It is vital that we take reports of cyber-bullying as seriously as reports of traditional bullying.

Outdoor activity and the natural environment

There has been growing concern that children are spending less time playing in the outdoors. A variety of reasons have been proffered for this, including risks about safety and increased traffic on the roads (Lester & Russell, 2010). Tovey (2007) also describes decreased adult tolerance of outdoor play, citing an example whereby a nursery had to reduce the time they spent with the children outdoors as neighbouring residents had complained about the noise. Examples such as this are hopefully few and far between.

A particularly broad influence, however, is likely to be that children's lives have become far more institutionalised, for example, with the introduction of breakfast and after-school clubs, some children may spend up to 10 hours in care outside of the home, leaving little time for free play (King & Howard, 2012).

Children gain a great deal from being in the natural environment, and this is reflected in the increased emphasis on outdoor play in early years curricula initiatives and the growth of the Forest School movement. These initiatives place particular emphasis on children being able to explore and learn from their natural environments, which, where possible, should contain: wild spaces and spaces for hiding; large spaces for running and moving; and hills and elevated spaces for rolling, climbing and jumping. Children are encouraged to explore independently and, in the Forest School movement, it is not always necessary for children to be in the sight of the school leader (Doyle, 2006).

This is an interesting concept, and can be difficult for some teachers to come to terms with, as being able to see children is often a principal means of ensuring their safety. A perception of freedom and not being under adult control contributes to the attraction of outdoor activity, however, and developing strategies to facilitate this is paramount.

The benefits of outdoor activity are many, and experiences are rich in opportunity for development across all domains. In the outdoors, children can move freely and energetically, with benefit to their motor skill development and overall physical health (Fjortoft, 2004). The outdoors is rich in sensory experiences, with sounds of different types and volumes, sensations such as feeling the wind or the warmth of the sun, and a variety of unreplicable colours and textures. Children will delight in observing the way that stones change colour when painted with water and will be equally in awe as the original colour returns. The opportunities for learning about shape, size and perspective are many.

In particular, however, being outdoors promotes a sense of wellbeing. Thompson *et al.* (2011) demonstrate that taking exercise in a natural environment often has a more positive impact on wellbeing than undertaking the same exercise indoors, and there are a variety of studies that demonstrate that at-risk or disaffected children and young people can benefit from intervention programmes based on outdoor activities, particularly in relation to building resilience, confidence and self-esteem (Davis-Berman & Berman, 2008). Being in the outdoors helps children to understand their identity and sense of self in the wider world and can lead to a more positive approach to future citizenship (Nutbrown & Clough, 2009).

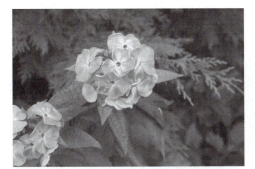

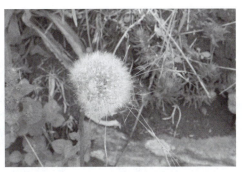

The natural environment is amass with unreplicable colour and texture throughout the year

Now that you have read the chapter

- Would you like to undertake training or further training in play?
  - Play training can be undertaken at vocational, applied or clinical levels.
  - Look up training opportunities in playwork, developmental and therapeutic play or play therapy on the internet and establish if there is anything available in your area.
- Talk to your colleagues about play. Discuss the different reasons that you think it is important for children's development.
- Reflect on the types of play materials and experiences you provide in your setting. Do you think they offer children the opportunity to utilise and develop their play skills?
- Undertake some one to one play sessions and some group play sessions.
  - How did your experiences differ?
  - What do you think are the benefits and limitations of each?

Useful further reading

Cowie, H. (2012) *From Birth to Sixteen: Children's Health, Social, Emotional and Linguistic Development* (London: Routledge).
This is a very useful book and essential reading for all children's service professionals

Jennings, S. (1999) *Introduction to Developmental Playtherapy* (London: Jessica Kingsley Press).
A valuable book to outline the importance of embodied, projective and role play, relevant and accessible to any children's service professional.

Inclusive play practice

Introduction

> If I am to walk along a road, I need a pair of shoes; but there are those who need a wheelchair, or a pair of crutches, or a guide dog, or other things beside. These needs could be identified and met, and then, off we could all go together.
>
> Baroness Warnock, 1986, cited in Abbott & Langston, 2005

Often, when we consider the concept of inclusivity our initial focus can too easily drift toward issues relating to disability. Two contrasting models of disability are presented in the literature – the medical model and the social model – and these have shaped the way in which we perceive and plan for difference and diversity in contemporary society.

The traditional medical model of disability tended to focus exclusively on the nature of any impairment and what made a child different. Emphasis was placed on diagnosis, causality and remediation, arguably seeing the impairment before seeing the child as an individual in their own right. Difference was seen as a barrier to ordinary services, and from a professional practice perspective children's needs were often seen as being best met by the provision of alternative rather than existing services. As is argued by Chapman (2010), if we think a solution to meeting the needs of those who are in some way different is to separate and segregate, then we send out a message that society is only really equipped and prepared to meet the needs of typically developing children.

In contrast, the social model of disability views the child first and foremost as an individual. Rather than solely focusing on the identification and assessment of a child's developmental limitations and provision for any additional needs, the social model seeks to identify and reduce potential limitations and barriers within society that may prevent access to ordinary services and life experiences. The social model celebrates diversity and difference, and seeks to promote authentic inclusive practice. It recognises our individual strengths and weaknesses within the context of culture and society.

Arguably, a move toward the social model of disability has led to a change in thinking about inclusivity on a much larger scale. Inclusive practice is an important component of a wider move toward enabling environments and the development of positive relationships that ensure that all children are given the opportunity to reach or exceed expectation, fulfil early promise and develop potential. It is founded on the notion of participation, fulfilment and success (West-Burnham, 2008). While physical and mental disability or illness can pose as a significant challenge for individuals, their families and service providers, inclusive practice is about far more than this. It emphasises that we all have individual needs and the right for these individual needs to be met within a barrier-free society. Through constant professional reflection, inclusive practice is about reducing attitudinal, environmental or institutional barriers to encourage feelings of belonging and self-worth (Chapman, 2010).

It is important, however, that we take a balanced view. The assessment of individual needs, understanding causality and the impact that difference, diversity or adversity can have on behaviour, development and life experience is vital to the provision of quality services.

Policy relating to play and inclusion

The Every Child Matters agenda (DfES, 2004b) specifies that its five main aims for all children are that they: enjoy good physical and mental health and have a healthy lifestyle; stay safely protected from harm and neglect; enjoy and achieve, getting the most out of life; make a positive contribution to society; and achieve economic wellbeing, free from the disadvantages of poverty. The Children's Plan (DCSF, 2007) described how play was a key to achieve many of these aims, and significant funds were dedicated to ensure adequate play provision and the training of a skilled play workforce. This was reflected in the Play Strategy (DCSF, 2008), which specified that

> Play is not only a vital part of the way children enjoy their childhood, but is central to all the *Every Child Matters* outcomes. Play is essential for children's good physical and mental health and development. Through taking risks whilst playing, they also learn how to manage risk – helping them to stay safe. Play develops learning skills, central to achievement, and is essential for the development of the skills that children and young people need as they become adults and move on in education or into work.
>
> DCSF, 2008, p. 4

Although the funding associated with the play strategy was lost in England as part of austerity measures following the formation of the coalition government in 2010, the message from these documents and the measures already put in place was clear: all children need and have the right to access appropriate play provision. A number of significant achievements relating to play provision were made across children's services, for example, emphasising play within the early years school curriculum, provision for play within Sure Start centres, guidelines relating to the play of children visiting parents in prison and the need for play strategies to meet the diverse needs of all children. Measures were designed to ensure that play places were attractive, welcoming, engaging and accessible for children and young people, including children who are disabled, children of both genders, and children from minority groups in the community (DCSF, 2007).

The legal right of all children to play is reflected in Article 31 of the United Nations Convention on the Rights of the Child (the UNCRC) (Davey & Lundy, 2011). It also features in English legislation in the Disability Discrimination Act (the DDA) (2004) and the Special Needs and Disability Act (2001), and in the National Service Framework for Children, Young People and Maternity Services (Department of Health, 2005).

In Wales, the Welsh Assembly Government has maintained an emphasis on the importance of play provision across children's services, and argues that providing for play is one of the most important things we can do to improve children's health and wellbeing, and that it is essential to development (Welsh Assembly Government, 2012). Not only does the Assembly promote the value of play across children's services, including in hospital, school, recreational and social care settings, but they also emphasise the promotion of play to ensure that all of society becomes aware of its importance. Crucially, they highlight how offering adequate opportunity to play not only enhances the development of all children across domains but also has the potential to increase children's resilience, enabling them to meet the challenge of difference and diversity (Welsh Assembly Government, 2011). This echoes the thoughts of Fearn and Howard (2011), which will be presented in Chapter 7.

Central to policy relating to children's play, however, is the notion of freedom, choice and control. As is pointed out by King and Howard (2012), definitions of what is means to play in legislation across the United Kingdom and within the UNCRC are based on a definition of play being where activities are freely chosen, personally directed and intrinsically motivated, what children and young people do when they follow their own ideas and interests, in their own way and for their own reasons. As these authors argue, given that children are spending an increasing level of time under adult supervision within the institutional triangle of the home, school and out of school club, we need to make a concerted effort to ensure that feelings of choice and control in play are upheld. This is the case regardless of difference or diversity.

King and Howard (2012) compared children's perceived levels of choice in their play across home, playground and out of school club settings. Interestingly, the club setting staffed by trained professionals who were knowledgeable about play was where children's choice levels were highest. This supports the notion that all children's service professionals would benefit from training in the facilitation of choice and control and the maintenance of play flow. We talk about this in Chapter 4 and, indeed, as we have tried to exemplify throughout this book, these key features of play are those that elevate it above and beyond mere fun and recreation. These are the inherent characteristics of play that render it such a valuable mechanism for enhancing development across domains (Howard, 2010c). Facilitating children's choice and control about what, where and with whom to play also meets the demands of an inclusive environment where practice needs to be flexible and person-centred so that it respects and responds to individual needs (Chapman, 2010).

Difference and diversity in children's play

As was highlighted in Chapter 2, children's play tends to follow a developmental pattern from a social and cognitive perspective. Socially, play progresses from activity that is relatively solitary to that which is a shared and co-operative experience. In line with theories of cognitive development (e.g. Piaget, 1951), play also tends to begin with activity that involves the senses and an understanding of the physical self, through to activity that involves symbolic action, pretence and an understanding of other's perspectives. Finally, play reflects children's increasing appreciation of rule-based activities. This typical pattern of development in children's play can be influenced (temporarily or permanently) as a result of difference and diversity or adverse experience.

From an ecological systems perspective (Valsiner, 2000), all of children's life experiences will be different in some ways and, as professionals, we are obliged to consider children's development and behaviour in light of what we know about their physical, social and intellectual condition as well as their social or familial circumstance. Some particular areas of difference and diversity, however, are now considered in the section that follows, with a particular emphasis on the implications of the knowledge we can gain from research and theory, in relation to professional play practice.

Play, gender and cultural context

Gender and cultural context are unlikely to impact on the development of children's play skills. Although the content of their play may differ, both boys and girls across all cultural contexts demonstrate progression through sensory, symbolic and role types of play – indeed, this repertoire of play skills may be seen as universal (Sheridan, Howard & Alderson, 2010).

In relation to gender differences exhibited in play, research demonstrates quite consistently that boys tend to participate in more physical rough and tumble activity than girls, and this finding is replicated in studies of animal behaviour (Jarvis, 2006). These findings have been used to support the proposition that this type of play behaviour may be biologically pre-programmed or serve some kind of evolutionary function. However, studies of parenting behaviour also demonstrate that parents (and more often fathers) are more likely to engage in this type of physical play with their male children, lending support to theories that suggest that gendered behaviour is a result of social learning (Bussey & Bandura, 1999).

In terms of professional play practice, Smith (2010) makes the interesting observation that perhaps one reason why this type of play is often perceived as problematic (and is subsequently curtailed) in primary school playgrounds is because staff tend to be female and have had less experience with this type of activity. This proposition could also be extended to a number of other children's services, particularly care-oriented contexts, where female–male staff ratios are often biased. In a similar way to our discussion regarding maintenance of the play flow more generally in Chapter 4, Smith highlights that of importance to professionals here is that they understand the cues to playful rather than real fighting, for example, there is a playful expression; that the activity does not draw the attention of peers; that blows are light and do not involve maximum strength; that there are signs of turn-taking; and that there are no obvious signs of conflict.

Gender differences have also been found in children's play preferences or toy choices. From as early as 2 years, research has demonstrated that boys tend to favour construction activities and wheeled toys whereas girls are more likely to choose dolls, dressing up or role play (Zosuls, 2009). Similarly to gendered patterns of rough and tumble play, the early onset of gendered toy preferences, however, can also be explained by the nature of parent–child interaction and interaction during play with peers (Rogoff, 2003) as well as by the reinforcement of gender roles via the media and through gift purchases made by friends and relatives (Fisher-Thompson, 1993). In professional practice, therefore, it is important that we are aware of gender stereotypes and the potential for these to shape the experiences we provide for the children in our care.

Just as a child's understanding of gender roles may be reflected in the content of their play, so too can we observe the modelling of cultural norms. Mahima, from Jammu in India, describes how Hindu culture was reflected in the wedding game she and her friends would play with their Barbie dolls. While the theme of marriage and weddings may be common to other cultures, here we are able to see how the finer details of the event permeated the play content. (See Scenario A.)

Scenario A

In Hindu culture, the bride goes to the groom's house only after getting married. So, in my play with Barbie dolls, my Barbie got married and went to her husband's house after the ceremony.

At the ceremony, my Barbie was dressed in red as it's an auspicious colour. She was made to wear a red lehanga (gown) with an odhnai (veil), which was stitched by my mother. She was heavily accessorised with artificial jewellery, Mom's lipstick and bindi. I remember calling all my friends from the neighbourhood, throwing a party at my home in the garden as a reception. There were invitees from the groom's side too (some boys from our neighbourhood) who had to be looked after well. The boy's side got their groom, a

GI Joe doll, who was dressed in a golden outfit and a red turban. We got all our toys to pretend to cook food for the reception. The food was chips, chocolates, coke, cookies, and if Mom was generous, some samosas and pakoras. I also remember inviting our parents to attend the wedding function. We used to put bedsheets on the lawn for everybody to sit and a few chairs as well.

After receiving the guests, the groom and bride were made to sit on colourfully decorated small chairs (that we got from my Mom's nursery school). All my friends used to sing songs and dance around. It was known as a sangeet (singing and dancing) ceremony. After a while the bride and groom used to take rounds of fire (we pretended there was a fire there). My brother was the 'pandit' (priest who performs the wedding ceremony). Then Barbie and GI Joe were called as husband and wife.

I remember sending my bride home with the groom (who lived in my neighbourhood). I said goodbye to Barbie (hugging and feeling bad to leave her). After a month or so I would take Barbie back because, as a child, I wanted to be apart from my doll for only a short time but I wanted it to also be realistic and feel that she had gone to her new life.

As is argued by Sheridan, Howard and Alderson (2010), it is also important that we consider how in some cultures toys such as dolls hold particular spiritual or ceremonial significance and may not be used for play in the ways we might expect. Indeed, historically, dolls and small animal toys for children's play in Islamic societies were made without eyes, noses or mouths as the depiction of facial features on such items was not permitted under religious law. In contemporary society, there are differences in the way toys such as Barbie dolls look, and are marketed across cultures. For example, the way in which the Westernised Barbie doll is dressed and marketed is very different from the way in which she is dressed and marketed in Islamic societies (where she is called a Fullah doll). Whereas the body shape of the Westernised Barbie is adult, the body of the Fullah doll is childlike; and while Barbie has blonde hair and pale skin, the Fullah doll has dark hair and brown skin. The Westernised Barbie has a vast array of modern clothes in line with current fashion trends, whereas the Fullah is dressed in the Hijab, has a prayer mat and a much more modest and simplistic collection of alternative outfits. Of importance to our professional practice here is that we are not only ensure that culturally diverse products are available, but that also we appreciate that the way in which the products look and are marketed conveys messages about cultural norms and values.

Importantly, in terms of accessing service provision, Alharbi (2012) reminds us of crucial differences in parenting behaviours between individualistic and collective cultures and the role of religion in matters such as health care, child development and education. She describes how Muslim parents may not make decisions about the care of their child alone, but that rather this would likely involve the immediate and extended family as well as the community. In addition, she describes how some Muslims may be disinclined to seek health care services such as play therapy because of their belief that Islam should provide all of the answers to personal and family problems.

Smith (2010) describes in detail the ways in which children's play varies across culture in relation to factors such as the time that is made available to play; the attitudes a particular culture may have toward the value of play; the physical environment and materials available for play; and how others interact with children as they play, in particular the role of parents and other adults. All of these things are important considerations for professional play practice and, through observation and reflection, it is vital that our practice is respectful and well-informed.

Play and disability

As is outlined by Herbert (2003), there has been much debate (often political) about which terminology we should adopt when describing children who are atypically developing. With reference to the World Health Organisation, Herbert provides the following useful definitions (p. 4):

- *impairment* – any loss of normal psychological, physiological or anatomical structure or function;
- *disability* – the limitation of personal activity consequent upon impairment, any restriction or lack of ability (resulting from an impairment) to perform an activity in the manner or within the range considered normal;
- *handicap* – the resulting personal or social disadvantage resulting from an impairment or disability that limits or prevents the fulfilment of a role that is normal (according to age, gender, social or cultural factors) for that individual.

The DDA (2005) defines disability as 'a physical or mental impairment which has a substantial and long-term adverse effect on a person's ability to carry out day-to-day activities'. Day-to-day activities are defined as: mobility; manual dexterity; physical coordination; continence; ability to lift; speech, hearing, vision; memory or ability to concentrate, learn or understand; understanding of risk or physical danger. Impairment may lead to disability that is moderate to profound. Children may have a disability that is physical, sensorial (involving hearing or vision), cognitive, behavioural or emotional. In many cases, impairment may be complex, extending across two or more of these areas. Indeed, often impairment in one developmental domain may lead to, or at least appear associated with, impairment in another. For example, while the development of early speech sounds progresses within normal levels in a child who is deaf up until around 9 months of age, the rate at which vocabulary develops subsequent to this can be significantly reduced, at around 200 words at around 4 years compared to 2,000 in a typically developing child (Herbert, 2003).

As has been noted elsewhere (e.g. Porter *et al.*, 2008), because of these complexities it can be difficult to meaningfully categorise types of disability for discussion. In his innovative and insightful book written from the perspective of a child with complex needs, Orr (2003) reminds us that regardless of the nature or extent of any impairment, enabling a degree of choice and autonomy should be central to our practice. With the best of intentions, these things can often be inadvertently overlooked, and those with

Table 6.1 The characteristics and potential implications of some types of impairment for play and play practice

Impairment	Potential characteristics	Potential challenges in relation to play	Practice foci
ADHD	Inattentiveness and/or hyperactivity and impulsivity	General delay in progress of play skills Shorter play episodes Failure to complete play activities Underdeveloped imaginative play Difficulty understanding or following rules Problems with social relationships Poor concentration Forgetfulness Low understanding of danger and risk	Outdoor activity can be particularly beneficial to expend energy Employ focusing techniques and wind-down time Use clear and simple boundaries Model and extend child's self-directed play Encourage turn-taking and social interaction Limit materials to avoid overstimulation Encourage the completion of short activities
ASD	Difficulties with social relationships, communication and imagination Often but not always, intellectually impaired	Engagement in ritual repetitive behaviours Social isolation Preference toward routine and familiarity Low levels of pretend/imaginative play Anger or frustration Hyper- or hypo-sensorial sensitivity Difficulty understanding nonverbal cues, other people's point of view, risk and danger, jokes or humour	Develop clear and simple boundaries, reflect and track play activity Use alternative communication techniques Focus on relationship development Encourage ways of experiencing and understanding the self to encourage progress toward symbolism and pretence

	Characteristics	Effect on play	Strategies
Down's Syndrome	Distinct facial characteristics Delayed development in speech, fine and gross motor skills and cognition Poor muscle tone Susceptibility to heart defects, vision and hearing problems	Slower play progress related to delay with gross and fine motor skills Repetition of familiar play activities Problems manipulating small play materials Lower attention span	Model and extend child's self-initiated play Encourage turn-taking and group work Develop social skills, confidence and independence Support physical play and understanding of the self Consider larger small world toys
Vision and hearing impairments	Fully or partially blind or deaf	More time needed to make sense of the environment, particularly for blind children Pretend play may develop more slowly and be less imaginative Preference may be toward solitary activity Relationships may be difficult to establish	Maximise use of available senses to learn about self and the environment Encourage turn-taking and interaction Support physical play to develop balance and co-ordination
Speech impairments	Difficulty producing speech sounds Stuttering Language delay Language disorder	Limited vocabulary and sentence construction Difficulty communicating with others Pretend play may be more slow to develop Prefer solitary play Relationships difficult to establish	Create a language-rich environment Play activities to expand vocabulary and language Model and extend simple play scripts Encourage turn-taking and group work

Table 6.1 Continued

Impairment	Potential characteristics	Potential challenges in relation to play	Practice foci
Cerebral palsy	Stiffness, uncontrollable movements, poor co-ordination and balance, potential language and intellectual impairment. Susceptibility to learned helplessness	Difficulties with mobility and accessing materials. Early sensory and self-play underdeveloped. Problems manipulating small play materials. Low confidence in the self, own ability to make choices and to impact on the environment	Focus on confidence and esteem. Support physical activities. Encourage sensory experiences. Consider larger small world toys. Enable choice and activities to demonstrate cause and effect
Dyspraxia	Difficulty executing fine and gross physical movement. Short-term memory problems. Hyper- or hypo-sensorial sensitivity	Early sensory and self-play underdeveloped. Problems manipulating small play materials. Immature drawing skill and less imaginative play. Underdeveloped pretend play scripts. Difficulty following instructions	Support physical activities. Encourage sensory experiences. Model and extend simple play scripts. Consider larger small world toys
Sensory integration disorders	Body has difficulty managing sensorial information. This could include difficulty in regulating information; filtering out what is not needed; discriminating information and/or the ability to plan	Avoidance of sensory activities due to confusion or feelings of overstimulation. Underdeveloped symbolic or pretend play. Repetitive simple play. Difficulty manipulating play materials or co-ordinating the self in gross motor play	Support sensory play activity with particular emphasis on discrimination. Avoid overuse of materials with multiple sensory outputs. Encourage and support physical activities to improve balance and co-ordination. Model and extend simple play scripts. Maximise play opportunities that build

Condition	Characteristics	Impact on play/development	Support strategies
	movements. There may be muscle weakness and co-ordination problems		on individual strengths to encourage a positive sense of self
Learning difficulties	No single profile, difficulty can affect one or many areas of learning, including: motor skills, language problems, maths/reading difficulties and auditory/visual processing problems	Largely dependent on the type and extent of the difficulty May be a general delay in the development of play skills and also lower confidence and self-esteem	Ensure a full understanding of the nature of the difficulty Maximise play opportunities that build on individual strengths to encourage a positive sense of self
Spina bifida	Muscle weakness Paralysis of lower body Curvature of the spine Bladder and bowel control problems Hydrocephalus Learning difficulties (all to varying degrees)	Difficulties with mobility and accessing materials Frequent hospitalisation or the need the need to deal with a shunt or catheterisation Delayed development of play skills Low confidence	Support physical activities to learn about self and environment Develop a positive sense of self and confidence in abilities Consider emotional support in relation to ongoing medical needs
Cystic fibrosis	Build up of secretions affecting lungs and digestive system Problems may include chest infections, coughs, stomach upsets and diarrhoea and poor weight gain	Frequent hospitalisation or need to attend daily physiotherapy or occupational therapy sessions Under-confident or lacking in esteem Potential delay in play skills as a result of the above	Encourage physical activities to support healthy lung functioning Develop a positive sense of self and confidence in abilities Consider emotional support in relation to ongoing medical needs

impairments are often given few opportunities to exercise choice due to low expectations and over-protection (ODI, 2010). Simple strategies, however, may involve the use of switches and buttons, communication boards, activity labels or simply ensuring a choice of activity, materials or equipment is available. As is argued by Doherty (2009), enabling choice and control ensures that children with impairments remain actively engaged in play activity, rather than passive participants reliant on adult direction.

We now consider three particular disabilities in relation to play and development: cerebral palsy, dyspraxia and autism. Space limits our ability to cover a wide range of disabilities with this level of detail, and thus, the accompanying table summarises a further (although not exhaustive) selection, outlining any potential impact on play and development along with suggestions for professional practice.

Cerebral palsy

The play patterns of children with motor impairments are likely to be influenced by a limited or reduced ability to interact with materials. For example, they may need support in accessing or utilising equipment or the play space may require alteration in order to accommodate their needs. Alternative types of play materials may also be required. Two such impairments are cerebral palsy and dyspraxia. Children who have cerebral palsy, a neurological disorder affecting movement, often suffer limb stiffness, uncontrollable movements, poor co-ordination and balance. Children with this condition may also suffer cognitive and linguistic impairment, but this is not always the case. Some children with cerebral palsy may be confined to a wheelchair whereas others may be able to walk with a frame or unaided.

The common motor symptoms of the condition may have implications for children's ability to engage effectively in early physical and sensory play, which is crucial to their developing sense of self. Opportunities to find out about themselves and the world around them through experiences involving sight, sound, taste, smell and touch are essential. Children can be encouraged to move in as many ways as they can, and to use and stretch their muscles in playful ways, for example, through musical and movement activities involving light, feathers or scarves. With an understanding of the self and confidence in their own abilities, children may move on to play with objects, using these in symbolic play, although difficulties with muscle tone and co-ordination may mean that materials that are larger and easier to grip are needed. For example, palm-sized cars may be more appropriate than the smaller matchbox versions.

It has been noted that children with cerebral palsy can be particularly at risk of learned helplessness, not behaving in a way that reflects their true ability because they feel unable to impact on the world around them (Ahonen-Eerikäinen, Lamont & Knox, 2008). Providing ample opportunity for children with cerebral palsy to interact with materials (physical, sensorial and symbolic) enables them to experience cause and effect. These types of play experiences are particularly useful for increasing resiliency, self-confidence and self-esteem, and subsequently help to maximise development across domains.

Dyspraxia

Children with dyspraxia have difficulties planning and executing physical movements, but have normal reflexes and muscle tone. Difficulties can involve gross motor, fine motor and linguistic skills to differing degrees, or a combination of these things. Children may also suffer from over- or under-sensitivity to sensory experiences and short-term memory problems, making remembering routines or instructions quite difficult (Kirby, 2006). Increased awareness among parents and practitioners now means that early signs such as a delay in reaching locomotor milestones, difficulties with feeding or frequent bumps and falls can be early signals prompting assessment. Of principal importance is awareness and understanding of the condition by professionals and peers, in order to prevent the onset of any emotional trauma or avoidance of particular play activities owing to embarassment, low confidence or esteem.

Children with dyspraxia may display immature drawing and be less inclined toward imaginative and creative play (Dyspraxia Foundation, 2012). Similarly to the child with cerebral palsy, they can be encouraged to become confident in their sense of self through physical and sensory activities. The nature of the activity may depend on whether they are under- or over-sensitive to this type of experience. Practitioners should seek to provide opportunities that enable children to learn about their competencies in relation to balance, for example, using balance bicycles or a balance board. Through extending and modelling during or after a child's own directed play, a practitioner may encourage imaginative activities. Puppets can be a useful way to achieve this, being relatively easy to handle and integrate into drama and storytelling. Again, larger or easy-grip toys can be encouraging and prevent feelings of frustration.

Autism

Reduced inclination toward creative and imaginative play and poor co-ordination are also signs that a child may have an autistic spectrum disorder (ASD). Both, however, are distinct conditions, with diagnosis for ASD involving triadic assessment with regard to social relationships, communication as well as imaginative activity (Wing & Gould, 1979). Motor co-ordination difficulties (such as those exhibited by children with dyspraxia) are most often found in children diagnosed as having Asperger's syndrome, which sits at the high-functioning end of the ASD. They may have relatively normal or high levels of intelligence and fewer problems with speech, but find it difficult to read and respond appropriately to social cues in communication.

There have been many empirical studies about the play of children on the ASD, many consistently demonstrating their lower levels of imaginative or pretend play (Jarrold, 2003). Children with autism often demonstrate more solitary play and play episodes that are shorter in duration (Eisele & Howard, 2012). A further characteristic of the condition is a tendency toward ritualised or repetitive behaviours, and this is often viewed as problematic and requiring remediation. Indeed, it has been proposed that ritual repetitive behaviour restricts children's engagement in other forms of activity, limiting the development of their social and symbolic play skills (Roeyers & Van Berkelaer-Onnes, 1994). Wing and Gould (1979), however, suggest that ritualised or repetitive behaviours may take the place of imaginative activities in autistic children.

Howard and Eisele (2012) studied the ritual repetitive behaviour of children with autism from the perspective of play, and found that in many cases episodes contained characteristics commonly associated with play such as enjoyment, laughter, energy, concentration and persistence. This work supports the view that perhaps we too often seek to mould the play behaviour of children with ASD into that which looks typical. In doing so, as we have argued throughout this book, we may lose sight of what it actually means to play. Luckett *et al.* (2007) strongly oppose the teaching of play skills, however, maintaining that it is possible to encourage children with ASD toward new experiences through playful engagement.

The success of such an approach can be seen in the child-led methods involved in relationship-based approaches to ASD intervention such as Intensive Interaction (Hewett & Nind, 2005) and Floortime (Greenspan, 2003). Both of these approaches, like non-directive play therapy (Axline, 1969), follow the child's lead, maintaining play flow to develop a warm and nurturing relationship. With this secure base, there is then scope to model new behaviours and experiences, giving children opportunity to develop their play repertoire.

A useful tool to inform practice in relation to which new experiences a child may be ready for in relation to the development to social skills, communication and symbolic play is the Westby Scale, details of which are provided in Chapter 7.

Play, sickness and hospitalisation

Illness has the potential to impact quite significantly on children's play, particularly if a child is sick for a long period of time or has to undergo hospital treatment. Even a child who has a minor temporary illness, such as a cold or a stomach upset, may not play in the ways that they usually do, perhaps preferring quieter activities or activities that are less socially or cognitively demanding. Changes in a child's behaviour and play activity are often quickly noted by observant teachers or classroom assistants, who might comment to parents at home time that their child does not seem to have been themselves. Change in play behaviour as a result of minor short-term illness can often be explained by the fact that fighting the illness makes a child tired and less inclined to set themselves complex challenges, preferring instead to take comfort in play activities they feel confident in and perhaps can complete without having to leave their bed or the sofa. The play of children with a minor temporary illness will return to its normal path as soon as they feel well.

For other children, illness may be long-term and in need of regular treatment, for example, eczema, asthma, diabetes or haemophilia. As is stated by Herbert (2003), children with chronic illness can be more susceptible to behavioural, cognitive, social and emotional difficulties. These are not attributable to the illness itself, but rather are a result of issues within the wider social context, for example, missing time at school; the quality of friendships and peer relations; any reduction in confidence and esteem; and disrupted play or leisure activity. Practitioners working with children who have these types of condition should carefully monitor behaviour in order to ensure long-term health and happiness.

As play is so important for developing confidence, relationships and a positive sense of self, particular care and attention must be paid to ensuring the promotion of a broad repertoire of play activities. Supporting the play of a child with a long-term illness requires us to make professional judgements with regards any potential risk associated with an activity in relation to a child's health condition, for example, whether chosen sensory play materials are likely to act as an irritant for a child with eczema or asthma.

This does not mean that a child cannot engage in an activity, only that materials and activities must be carefully selected and planned in accordance with individual needs. A child with chronic asthma might participate in a music and movement activity, but perhaps this may need to be shorter and involve small-scale rather than gross motor movements. A child with chronic eczema on their hands might complete foot rather than hand painting and enjoy dry rather than wet sensory materials (e.g. cotton wool balls, pasta, rice and cereals rather than shaving foam or cornflour 'gloop').

Some activities may simply be planned for enjoyment in the here and now, whereas others may have specific developmental objectives (for the being and becoming elements of play, see Chapter 1). When particular developmental outcomes are planned, coming up with alternatives to suit individual needs is often easier if we simply remember to ask ourselves 'what do I want the child to gain from this activity?' and 'how else could this be achieved'?

Management of risk and safety are further amplified when considering play for children in hospital. Play specialists in hospital environments must consider not only the health of each individual child, but also the health of all other children on the ward as well as general infection control. At a basic level this might necessitate frequent cleaning of toys and the surfaces within the play environment, and choosing materials that are disposable or easy to clean and less likely to harbour germs. In some hospitals, certain materials such as the use of cornflour 'gloop' or shaving foam must first be approved by the pharmacy team.

When a child is hospitalised they face many challenges, such as separation from friends and carers, a new and potentially unfamiliar and frightening environment, disruption to their usual routine as well as the prospect of treatment, surgery and the discomfort associated with their illness. The need for children to have access to appropriate play provision during a hospital stay is reflected in governmental policy and practice. Most children's wards, especially those in larger hospitals, will now have a play room and a team of play professionals. This may comprise playworkers, professionals trained in hospital play, and developmental and therapeutic play specialists. Some teams may also include trained child counsellors, child psychotherapists or play therapists.

Play in this context serves a variety of important functions. Being able to participate in familiar activities can help to make children feel more comfortable in the environment. It affords a sense of autonomy and control, and it makes children feel at ease and more able to cope with separation from family and friends. Using puppets and dolls, procedures can be modelled and children can see, touch and talk about the medical equipment they are likely to experience. This has been shown to reduce anxiety in both the child and their carer (Fincher, Shaw & Ramelet, 2012). Through story telling and story making, children can be prepared for the consequences of treatment and how they may feel after it has taken place (both physically and emotionally), and in the safety of playful activity they may be more likely to talk and ask questions (Li & Lopez, 2008).

Play can also serve as a distraction should a child need to undergo painful treatment, for example, the use of bubbles, music or interactive electronic games. It can also, of course, relieve boredom for those needing a long-term stay. Children facing a long-term

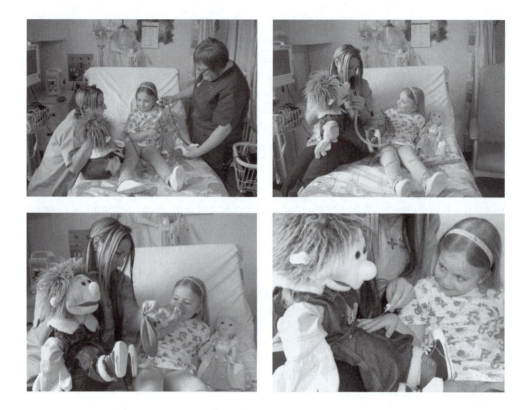

hospital stay, complex surgery or the diagnosis of an acute, chronic or fatal condition may be particularly susceptible to emotional trauma. In these cases, a trained counsellor or therapist might also use play to enable children to communicate and manage their feelings (McMahon, 2009). Children recover more quickly from illness and medical procedures if they are given the opportunity to play, and for this reason, along with the play team, paediatric physiotherapists, child nurses and occupational therapists may also use play when preparing children for a return to their home and regular routine.

> I originally trained as a Nursery Nurse, and for the last sixteen years I have been working on the children's ward. I am now completing a Master's degree in Developmental and Therapeutic Play. Puppets are a valuable part of my practice. I use them daily to welcome children, prepare them for theatre or simply as a way of encouraging children to talk with me.
>
> Lisa Morgan, Nursery Nurse and Play Leader, Morriston Hospital, Swansea

Play, adversity and emotional trauma

Just as play can help children to overcome the consequences of illness and hospitalisation, it also acts as a resource for those facing the consequences of adversity or emotional trauma. It is important, however, to consider the concept of resiliency – the resources children have available to them in order to meet life challenges – when we think about issues such as these. Whereas some situations or experiences might be easy to categorise as adverse or emotionally traumatic, for example, living in acute poverty, in a war zone or experiencing sexual abuse, the challenge of other events, such as divorce or growing up in foster care, may be more or less challenging depending on the resources a child has available to them.

Play can function at a preventative and remedial level. Recognising the capacity of play to prevent or minimise the potential impact of adversity or trauma highlights how crucial it is for all children's service professionals to have received training in play and to understand the characteristics inherent in play that render it such a powerful resource. From a remedial perspective, utilising play-based methods during counselling or psychotherapy can increase communication, reduce anxiety and help to form the therapeutic relationship. Allowing children to follow their own play process while tracking and reflecting on this during non-directive play can also be seen as therapy in itself, enabling children to share and make sense of their experiences. The way in which play can function in this respect is described in Chapter 5.

The value of play as a preventative resource for children facing adversity is exemplified in an analysis of case studies involving children's experiences of various non-normative crises by Howard and Fearn (2011). Their analysis focused on the reported experiences of children caught in the bombing of Beirut, children abandoned to the state system in Romania, and street children in Rio de Janeiro and Cali. Comparison across these different contexts showed that when given the opportunity, all of the children interacted with and influenced their environment through play, and this process provided a resource to meet the challenge of adversity.

The way in which play can prevent emotional trauma or the impact of adverse experience is also reflected in emotional literacy interventions such as SEAL (Social and Emotional Aspects of Learning), which focus on the development of a positive sense of self using group work and play-based activities (Humphrey et al., 2010). Services for children affected by domestic violence have also begun to include increased focus on play and emotional health, employing developmental and therapeutic play specialists to work alongside children in their play to improve confidence and esteem and to promote resilience. The freedom and autonomy in these play sessions enables a sense of control over an otherwise chaotic life and can help to minimise the impact of emotional trauma and the need for future mental health care.

Recent research also demonstrates that training in play for residential care staff can lead to their adoption of a proactive rather than reactive approach to children's care (Skeate, 2011). The same study also demonstrated that increased emphasis on play in the residential care environment impacted positively on the children's levels of happiness and emotional wellbeing.

In relation to looked-after children, recent foster care initiatives have also focused on training potential carers in relationship development and attachment, resiliency and the therapeutic potential of play in order to ensure they understand and are able to meet the needs of children with complex life histories or particular behavioural or emotional needs. Looked-after children, particularly those who have been in multiple care placements, may not have developed secure attachment bonds with their carers or may have had these attachment bonds broken as they have moved from place to place. Attachment problems and failure to develop a coherent life narrative can impact on the development of social, emotional and cognitive functioning (Greenberg, 2006).

Children with attachment difficulties may be emotionally and socially withdrawn and demonstrate developmental delay (Zeanah, Smyke, Koga & Carlson, 2005). They may play in ways that appear socially or cognitively immature or may show a strong preference toward or avoidance of particular play experiences because they have become associated with particular life events or they are unfamiliar to them. Here, children can be supported to play in ways they feel comfortable, with a particular emphasis placed on safe boundaries, consistency and unconditional positive regard. By enabling choice and control in play, confidence, esteem and trust can be promoted. A child may use their play to make sense of previous experiences and to try on and try out roles and emotions. Children are also likely to benefit from child-centred or non-directive play therapy (Bratton & Ray, 2000).

Meeting the needs of every child

Chapman (2010) suggests that good inclusive practice relies on us:

1. understanding what is meant by inclusivity;
2. understanding policy relating to inclusivity and the rationale for this;
3. working to eradicate stereotypes and prejudice;
4. developing a positive attitude;
5. developing respect;
6. promoting wellbeing for all;
7. engaging in constant assessment and reflection;
8. being prepared for change.

In a review of inclusion and the education of children through primary and secondary school years, MacBeath *et al.* (2006) indicate that to a large extent policy and practice appears to be working to meet these principles in that educators described an increase in positive attitude toward diversity and difference, a more thorough understanding of children's needs and various social benefits for all children involved. The report also highlights, however, complexity surrounding the identification and provision of the most appropriate support in relation to inclusivity (whether this is within standard mainstream services or through specialist, more segregated provision). As is argued by Abbott and Langston (2005), there are times when children will benefit from being with children who have similar needs and times when they will benefit from being among those who are different.

Notwithstanding that inclusivity is about the provision of high-quality enabling environments for all children, there remains a legislative requirement for us to identify and respond to needs requiring specific intervention or service provision. Needs might be physical, emotional, behavioural, intellectual or a complex combination of these (Herbert, 2003). The Children Act (1989) states that children have specific needs if they are unlikely to achieve or maintain (or have the opportunity to achieve or maintain) a reasonable standard of health or development without the provision of specified services, that their health or development is likely to be impaired or further impaired without the provision of such service or if they are disabled. Such services might include occupational therapy, individual learning or behavioural support, speech and language therapy, educational psychology services, counselling, mental health care or access to social work professionals.

Knowing when a child may be in need of additional support or specialist services as soon as possible is crucial and, as is described in Chapter 7, because during play children often function at their optimum level, it can provide a key way to evaluate physical, intellectual, emotional or behavioural needs. As is specified in the Children's Plan (DCSF, 2007), we should aspire to a proactive rather than reactive approach, it being better to prevent failure than to tackle a crisis at a later date. There are a number of useful measures of play and child development which, in combination with information from other sources, and informal observations, can provide a useful indicator as to whether or not referral for further needs assessment may be beneficial. An important part of our professional role is understanding the nature of inter-agency working and pathways for referral within the contexts in which we work.

Conclusion

Inclusive play practice means providing materials and opportunities that enable all children to benefit from all types of play, not only in relation to the longitudinal developmental potential such opportunities may offer but also in terms of the immediate benefits of play in the here and now. As well as reflecting on the types of play materials we are providing for the children in our care, a key component of our practice is enabling children's choice and autonomy. Provision is about more than play opportunities, it is about creating the conditions for play (Lester & Russell, 2010). It requires that we support children's ability to play, create opportunities for children to be playful, and understand that play is where children are able to exercise choice and control.

Now that you have read the chapter

- In what ways to difference and diversity impact on your practice?
  - Do you feel you know enough about the cultures of the children in your care?
  - Can you remember any times when culture has been reflected in the play of children with whom you work?
- Revisit the steps toward inclusivity suggested by Chapman (2010) in relation to your own play practice.
  - Do you and your colleagues have a shared understanding of inclusivity?
  - Can you identify any challenges in relation to inclusive play practice in your setting?
  - How might these be overcome?

Useful further reading

Chapman, L. M. (2010) *Inclusivity*. Available from: www.equalitytraining.co.uk
A brief but informative pamphlet describing factors associated with implementing inclusive practice.

Orr, R. (2003) *My Right to Play: A Child with Complex Needs* (Buckingham: Open University Press).
A wonderful book, outlining key issues surrounding inclusive play practice. Written from the perspective of a child with complex needs, this accessible text outlines professional practice issues within the context of real-life experience.

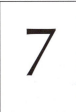

7 Observation and assessment through play

Aims of the chapter

- To highlight why play is such a useful medium for observation and assessment.
- To facilitate the development of key observation skills.
- To alert practitioners to the issue of bias and interpretation error.
- To present some basic observation strategies.
- To introduce some useful published measures.

Introduction

In Chapters 4 and 5 we discussed the important role of professionals in creating playful environments through the way that activities are presented and, crucially, the way that we interact with the children in our care. Observation and assessment were key components of this process, and you were provided with some practical suggestions as to how you could reflect on your practice. This chapter addresses the second important tenet of observation and assessment in play – that pertaining to the individual child. This chapter describes why observation and assessment are important for ensuring quality play experiences that suit individual children's needs, and also highlights the value of observing children at play as a means of identifying when additional professional assessment and intervention might be required. The chapter discusses why play is a particularly useful arena for monitoring children's development across domains, and presents a range of observation techniques. Caution about interpretation and bias in the observation process are also considered.

Observation and assessment as key elements of professional play practice

From an educational perspective in particular, there has been a great deal of debate in recent years about the extent to which we assess young children (Anning & Edwards, 2006). In particular, attention has been drawn to the limitations of standardised testing, such as how useful a predictor isolated standardised tests are of later achievement; whether an emphasis on standardised tests encourages assessment-driven practice (i.e. teaching to test); and whether the test process itself might subject young children to unnecessary emotional pressure and a vulnerability to feelings of failure or incompetence. Some practitioners have been able to resist testing practices whereas others, owing to governmental legislation, have not. Perhaps a common bugbear in relation to testing and assessment in the early years at school has been that the test results have not had any real added utility value. They have served as a formalised record of what teachers already know about the children in their care, collating but often repeating information already collected as part of good everyday professional practice.

There is no doubt, however, that observation and assessment are key elements of professional play practice across all of children's services. This is particularly the case for practitioners in an educational environment, who, given the extensive time they spend with children, are often in the best position to track developmental progress and to make important decisions about intervention and referral (Brassard & Boehm, 2008). Educational practitioners in particular, however, often report feeling uncomfortable or indulgent about allowing themselves time to observe children. This can be because they feel there are other more pressing requirements on their time or because they feel others (perhaps parents or colleagues) do not value observation as part of their professional role.

Being mindful as to the purpose of observation enables us to clearly articulate why it has such an important place in our professional practice. Observation, assessment and reflection serve to ensure that children are provided with the best possible play experiences, whether these be from an educational, therapeutic or recreational perspective. We also know that the best developmental trajectories for children are achieved when the need for additional support is identified as early as possible and, as such, observation also facilitates early intervention and referral to specialist children's services when this might be considered beneficial.

Epstein, Schweinhart, DeBruin-Parecki and Robin (2004) propose that the function of observation and assessment can be divided into that which pertains to the child (e.g. leading to early intervention or the tracking of children's developmental progress) and that which pertains to the environment or experiences being offered (e.g. leading to the identification of staff development needs or an evaluation of the activities and materials available).

The role of reflective practice and evaluation of the play environment has been covered in Chapters 3 and 4 of this text. The main focus of the current chapter relates to observation in relation to the development of children's play skills and evidencing children's development across domains during their play.

The value of play as a means of observing and assessing children's development

Children spend a great deal of their time engaged in play and, as such, it provides a natural opportunity to observe and document their development. Indeed, it has been said that play offers a window into children's developmental progress (Eisert & Lamorey, 1996; Oaklander, 1988; Stagnitti & Cooper, 2009). As we have argued earlier in the book, romanticised claims are often made about the value of play for children's development that are not particularly well supported by research evidence. While children certainly learn in a variety of different ways (for example, via observation, rote or direct instruction), using research evidence, we have demonstrated that there is something special about play that appears to enhance development across domains.

In Chapter 3 we described experimental studies that have repeatedly shown that when children perceive an activity as though it were play they demonstrate the following: deeper engagement; increased wellbeing; more purposeful problem-solving; and significantly improved task performance than when they perceive the *same activity* as not play. These findings not only provide us with evidence as to the value of play for children's development in general, but also the value of play as a means of observation and assessment.

Howard and Miles (2008, in Howard, 2010a) suggest a theoretical model of play that incorporates these findings, and propose that the beneficial effect of children approaching activities as play manifests in the provision of a protected environment where behavioural thresholds are lowered and, as a result, exploration, trial and error can occur. This is consistent with the view of Vygostky (1978) who commented that 'play creates a zone of proximal development [where] a child always behaves beyond his average age, above his daily behaviour . . . as though he were a head taller than himself' (1978, p. 102). Play offers a valuable means of assessment because children are more likely to perform to the best of their ability.

A similar view is put forward by Kelly-Vance and Ryalls (2008) when reviewing the benefits of play-based assessment. They argue that as well as being culturally sensitive, when observation and assessment occur in a natural play environment it is motivating and subsequently elicits the highest level of a child's functioning (p. 557).

Epstein *et al.* (2004) suggest that developmentally appropriate assessments for young children should: (1) not make children scared or anxious; (2) be completed during normal day-to-day activities; (3) be repeated across time and context; and (4) be sensitive to children's interests and attention span. Using these criteria, children's authentic play offers an excellent opportunity for observation and assessment.

Play offers a natural setting, a fear-free environment, it can be observed at various times and in various forms, and as play is chosen and directed by the child, interest and attention span are self-regulated. Use of the word authentic here, however, is key. In order to increase the reliability and validity of our play observations, it is important that the activities are seen by children to be as much like play as is possible. Activities must not be contrived, merely looking like play because they involve play materials (Walsh *et al.*, 2011). As we saw in previous chapters, encouraging children to see their activities as play can be maximised when we afford them autonomy and control.

Process, product and interpretation

Effective assessment in play should be ongoing, taking place at different times and across different activities. Whenever we reflect on our observations of children at play, we must consider the value of observing play as a process and, in particular, we should always be mindful of the dangers associated with interpretation. This is especially the case when considering play as a means of expressing emotion or play as an expression of lived experience. Play can be, but is not always, the re-enactment of experience. Play can be, but is not always, a reflection of our emotional state. Often, our interpretations of play can be based on what we, as adults, consider to be acceptable or normal forms of behaviour. We should bear in mind, however, that children often use play as a means of learning about the world and those around them and, as such, might not yet be bound by the same rules. Their play might therefore be scary, dark or sinister by adult interpretation, but it does not have this intent.

Smidt (2011) presents the case of 15-month-old Dov, who is given a doll when his new baby brother is born. Smidt reports that, at first, he holds the doll, rocks it in his arms, looks into its face and smiles. Six weeks later, he takes the doll out the pram, throws it to the floor and stamps on it. It is suggested that Dov is expressing feelings he is harbouring toward the new baby safely through play.

This interpretation might be right and it might be wrong. To make a more accurate judgement we would no doubt want to consider more details, for example, does this behaviour occur during all of the child's doll play or just during play with this specific doll? Does it really happen every time they play with the doll, or are we just more aware of the darker play? Are there any other signs that Dov might be troubled by the arrival of the new baby? Has their play or behaviour in general, changed in any other ways (for example, regression to less mature behaviour or a change in sociability)?

Misinterpretation can occur because we focus on the product of play (what is drawn, made or painted, or perhaps the theme of small world or role play) or because we make our interpretation out of context (observing just a small section of a play episode rather than the process in its entirety). These two interpretation errors are highlighted in the following case study examples. We are grateful to our colleagues for sharing these examples with us, and although we have likely made some mistakes in our documenting of the anecdotes, we hope we have captured the important messages contained within them.

Box 7.1 Exemplary anecdote

*The importance of observing process and product:
the child who always painted with black*

Read the following extract:

Andrew, aged 5, was a quiet child in class who would play alongside his peers and interact pleasantly when it was necessary, but he was never particularly chatty. His seemed to like playing alone, and would spend long periods of time building complex Lego models.

At the end of one day, the nursery assistant was busy unpegging all of the day's artwork from the drying line when she commented that Andrew had, yet again, painted his picture using nothing but black. It seemed to happen quite often, she noted. A serious discussion ensued between the teacher and the nursery assistant. Yes, staff had noticed his exclusive use of black paint before. Yes, Andrew was a particularly quiet child. Might Andrew's drawings be indicative of some kind of emotional upset? Was there anything going on in Andrew's home life that they were not aware of?

The class teacher decided to keep an eye on his artwork. Sure enough, a few days later, Andrew produced yet another black painting. Again, serious discussion ensued, only this time, the class teacher decided he would watch Andrew as he painted. At the start of the afternoon, the 'Dinosaurs', Andrew's class group, were told it was their turn to paint. With a lot of hustle and bustle, the children excitedly ran over to the art area and began choosing their materials. Andrew seemed to wait for the crowd to disperse before quietly and unhurriedly following. The teacher watched as he arrived at the art area. Andrew chose the only remaining pot of paint, and that paint was black! When offered different coloured paints, Andrew happily accepted.

The teacher was relieved at how easily Andrew's behaviour had been explained, and learned a valuable lesson as to the importance of observing both the process and product of play!

What are your thoughts on the extract? Can you identify any stereotypical bias? Can you think of any professional situations where you have made similar errors of judgement?

Box 7.2 Exemplary anecdote

The importance of considering behaviours in context: rough play with teddies

Read the following extract:

> The little girl, perhaps around 6 years old, settled into her seat on the plane clutching four small soft toys. She unfolded a blanket onto her lap and seated all of the toys in front of her. She studied them for a while, moving them carefully into their positions. She seemed quite mindful of the particular spacing between them. She took hold of two toys, a teddy with a protruding button nose and a softer, more squidgy-looking panda bear. For a few moments she felt them, pressing their noses in and out. Suddenly, with force, she took the button-nosed bear and pressed his face hard into the panda's face. Over and over again she forced his face down onto the face of the other teddy. Her fingertips were white and her hands shook with pressure. Her face was full of concentration and effort.

What are your initial thoughts on this observation?
  Continue reading:

> After quite a few minutes of pressing and squeezing, she moved the panda into a position in her cupped hand so that she was able to feel the back of his head. As she pressed the teddy, still concentrating hard on the process and applying considerable force, she looked at, and felt, the back of the panda's head. A small glimmer of a smile or a satisfied expression appeared on her face when she saw the protruding shape of the bear's nose on the back of the panda's head as she pressed.

What are your thoughts now? Have they changed in anyway? Why?
  Continue reading:

> The air steward came through the cabin, handing out headphone sets in small plastic bags. The little girl seated the teddies back into their positions on her lap and took a set of headphones. She opened the bag and took out the headphones, confidently plugging them in to the seat arm. Her attention remained on the very small plastic bag rather than the headset, however, and she gently stretched a larger hole in the bag with her fingers. Suddenly she picked up panda and 'walked' him over to the bag. She seemed to fight to squash the panda's head into the bag, struggling particularly with his ears, which were large and needed to be squeezed in order to fit. She squashed and squeezed with all her might to get the head to go into the small plastic bag. Again, her fingertips were white and her face was full of concentration and

effort. It took several minutes for her to squeeze the head enough for it to fit into the small plastic bag. Once it was done, she held the bag around the panda's neck with a clasped fist and lifted it up. Its arms and legs dangled while she turned the panda to view its head in the bag from all angles.

What are your thoughts about the little girl's behaviour?
   Continue reading:

As if suddenly satisfied that she had achieved her goal (getting the head into the bag, perhaps), the little girl then moved on to try out other body parts. She tried one leg, then two legs together. Then she tried the arm and then the other arm. When trying to get the second arm into the bag she accidentally made a hole in the bag with her finger. She poked her finger through, wiggling it back and forth. She looked deep in thought. She took out her finger and put the panda's arm through the bag instead. She made a further hole in the other corner of the bag and poked through the toy's second arm, 'dressing' the panda in the bag like a jacket. Panda was then 'walked' back to his seat on the girl's lap, dressed in his plastic jacket. Through the remainder of the flight all of the soft toys had a turn at wearing the jacket.

What are your thoughts now? Have they changed in any way? Why?

Developing observational skills

Observation and assessment in play can be structured, unstructured or a mixture of both. It can involve forms of documentation and observation schedules developed by practitioners themselves or it can involve the use of standardised measures. Standardised measures often have the benefit of being tested for their reliability and validity, which means they have been trialled with suitably representative samples of children over a period of time and that they reliably measure the behaviour(s) for which they were intended. Standardised measures are particularly useful for identifying when children might require additional support, for example, in the case of children on the autistic spectrum, children with hearing impairments or children with speech and language difficulties. In these cases, trained professionals utilise standardised measures, often comparing children against developmental norms, for diagnosis and to inform their decisions about intervention.

As this text is designed for professionals across a range of children's services, it is beyond our scope to discuss tests designed for the identification of particular needs. Rather, our aim is to equip practitioners with knowledge and skills they can utilise in their practice to make informed judgements about children's developmental progress and be alerted to when additional professional assessment and perhaps intervention might be required.

Often, reference to developmental norms or milestones is presented in a negative light, and is contrasted sharply to other more contextual forms of observation. While it is certainly true that children do not develop in a vacuum, it is also true that many aspects of children's development do follow a broad developmental pattern (Stagnitti & Cooper, 2009; Sheridan, Howard &Alderson, 2010). Being knowledgeable about patterns of child development, while at the same time appreciating that children develop within a social and cultural context, offers the most pragmatic and useful professional position. When making observations of any kind, it is important that we endeavour to be as objective as possible and that we are aware of any biases that might potentially influence our records or judgements. Children's behaviour can change simply because they are aware they are being observed, something that has come to be known as the Hawthorne Effect or experimenter bias in social science research. This can be remedied by observing as discreetly as possible and by ensuring children are comfortable with your presence by allowing a period of acclimatisation. Fawcett (1996) also asks us to be mindful of the ways in which our observations can be subtly influenced by pre-conceptions we as professionals might hold about children according to appearance, culture, religion, social class or gender. It is also important to be mindful of professional bias, for example, a little girl showing frustration and anger at not being able to complete a jigsaw puzzle could be attributed to many things. A professional working in a therapeutic context might be inclined to attribute the behaviour to an emotional issue; a professional in an educational context might attribute it to inferior spatial skills (perhaps influenced by a further bias of gender) and a hospital play professional might relate the frustration to the child's physical limitations associated with them having their arm in cast. In fact, it could be all of these things concurrently or none of them at all.

Observational techniques

Of key importance when deciding how to undertake observation and assessment is to clearly identify what you, as the professional, hope to achieve. What is the aim of your observation, and how will you collect the data you need in order to fulfil that aim? It is also important to remember that observation has most utility value when the process is ongoing and when a variety of documentation and assessment strategies are adopted (Brassard & Boehm, 2008). Undertaking a range of observations at different times will ensure that you make the most informed professional judgements possible and that you are less likely to make interpretation errors.

Whereas the observation and assessment designed to feed into staff development needs or evaluation of the play environment is likely to involve multiple children, observation designed to track developmental progress will almost exclusively involve a single child. Here your focus is on developing your professional knowledge of a particular child through detailed observations of them at play. There are a range of different observational techniques that you might consider adopting, and no approach is right or wrong. Experimenting with a range of approaches to find out what suits your professional needs as well as your personal preference is recommended.

Narrative techniques and diaries

Using narrative techniques such as a running records or anecdotal diary entries might appear to be the simplest form of observation, but they can be incredibly difficult. Diary entries tend to be overarching descriptions of events throughout a day or play session. They are often brief and, because they are generally written after the event, they rely on memory and may be more open to interpretation bias. They are useful, however, to remind us about particular one-off events that may have influenced a child's behaviour or to simply remind us of what happened the last time we met with a child. Brassard and Boehm (2008) suggest that the bias associated with retrospective recording can be avoided if we make our notes as soon as possible after the event, and that we clearly separate the facts about the event from our interpretive comments. (See Example 1 for a diary entry.)

Example 1: A diary entry

Child: Elisha
Age: 3 years 2 months
Date: Wednesday 15th October 2010
Entry by: Sandra (nursery manager)

Elisha's mum talked with me briefly this morning when she was dropping her in at the nursery. She said Elisha had not been sleeping very well for the past week or so. She said she was finding it hard to get her off to sleep and that she was also waking up more often than usual through the night. She asked how she was at nursery. I spoke to Elisha's key workers (Naomi and Claire). They said they had noticed Elisha was a little quieter than usual but that they thought this was because Ellie, her usual playmate, had been away from nursery on holiday for the past week.

NOTE: Monitor the situation and encourage alternative peer play. Let Mum know about Ellie's holiday as this might reassure her.

A *running record* is a descriptive account of everything that a child says and does in the context of their surroundings over a specified time period. Running records are less open to recall bias because they are completed in real time and do not rely on memory for events. Conducting observations in real time, however, can be associated with other limitations. When using a running record it is necessary to make judgements about what to write as invariably it is impossible to write down everything that we see. We also have to make decisions about the level of detail we choose to include.

Running records aim to capture action and speech as well as contextual detail, and for this reason they require intense concentration and are often time-restricted, say to around 15 minutes. The length of time we are able to focus on conducting a running record, however is very individual and may increase with experience. In addition, to solve the problem of performing observation and annotation concurrently, it can also be useful to develop a system of shorthand or abbreviation. (See Example 2 for a running record.)

Example 2: A running record

Date: Thursday 22nd September 2009
Time: 3.45–4.00pm
Activity: Craft table
Children present: Molly (M), David (D), Freya (F)
Adults present: Joyce (J)
Any target child or aim: encouraging Molly to take part in more messy activities
Observation made by: Sally (S)

Time	Notes
3.45	D and F quickly choose a large sheet of coloured paper and begin to cut pictures from magazines and stick these on
	J – 'would you like to come and stick Molly?'
	M nods and comes to sit at the table. She has her hands in her lap, occasionally she looks up to see what D & F are doing
3.48	J says 'what would you like to do Molly?'
	M shrugs and replies 'dunno'
3.52	J says 'I'm going to do some sticking like David and Freya'
	M continues to watch as J picks up her materials
	J asks if any of the children can find her a picture of a dog to stick on
	M says 'I'll find you one' and looks through the toy catalogue. She finds a picture of a soft toy dog and points it out to J.
3.55	J says 'can you cut it out for me Molly?'
	M responds 'I'll have a try'
	J – 'fab'
	M holds the scissors quite awkwardly and cuts roughly around the picture
3.58	J – says 'thanks' and Molly asks if she wants any other 'stuff' cut out
	J says that would be great
	M selects another soft toy and cuts this out, again roughly and with an awkward grasp on the scissors
	D cuts out a toy bike and passes it over to M and says 'you could have this one to stick on too if you like'
	M carefully takes the bike picture from D's gluey hand with her index finger and thumb, she kind of smiles but doesn't say anything. She places it down onto the table with the other soft toy she has cut. M asks J if she can go and do dress up now. J responds – 'course'

Notes: Molly was a little hesitant when Joyce asked if she'd like to join them at the craft table. She didn't seem that confident in using the scissors but had a try at cutting. She didn't do any gluing. Perhaps she will next time. I wondered if David offering her a picture he'd cut out made her self conscious, perhaps that was why she left the activity and went to the dress up area?

Diagrammatic techniques

Diagrammatic techniques can be a useful way of recording children's behaviour as it occurs across the playroom at large. Tracking children's movements using a playroom map allows us to observe a variety of things, for example, how quickly children move from one activity to the next; whether they always tend to move from one particular activity to another; and whether certain activity areas are preferred whereas others are neglected. Watching children's freely chosen activity using tracking can be a useful starting point for more detailed observation. For example, if a child tends not to engage with the messy play area, this might be introduced and their behaviour then observed. (See Example 3 for a tracking diagram.)

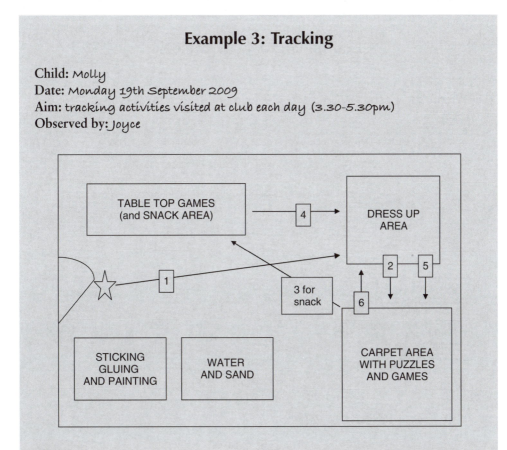

Example 3: Tracking

Child: Molly
Date: Monday 19th September 2009
Aim: tracking activities visited at club each day (3.30-5.30pm)
Observed by: Joyce

TABLE TOP GAMES
(and SNACK AREA)

DRESS UP
AREA

4

1

3 for
snack

2   5

6

STICKING
GLUING
AND PAINTING

WATER
AND SAND

CARPET AREA
WITH PUZZLES
AND GAMES

Notes:
Molly spent most time at the dress up area with Martha today. She briefly played with the garage and cars on the carpet twice, but only for a few minutes or so. She came to table top area for snack but didn't visit it when there were table top games. She didn't visit the messy play area.

An *activity clock* can provide a useful diagrammatic summary of how a child spends their time through a day or play session. The clock is divided into predefined time periods. In the case of the example provided below (adapted from West, 1996), a 30-minute play session is divided into six 5-minute segments. In the first inner ring, the social context of the play is recorded using an A if an adult is present, and then an M or an F for each other child involved (indicative of their gender). This social coding system can be further elaborated to indicate whether an adult or other children are merely present (by recording A, M or F), or present and interacting (coding AI, MI or FI). In the next ring, notes about the activity or type of play can be recorded, for example, small play with the farm or play with musical instruments. The outermost section can be used to write details of what was going on or comments the professional might wish to make. (See Example 4 for an activity clock.)

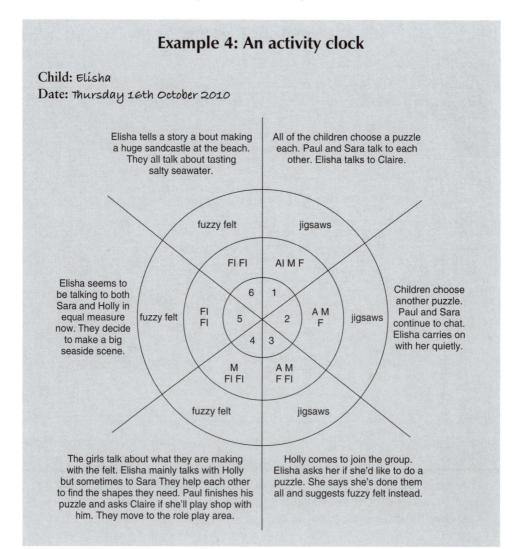

Example 4: An activity clock

Child: Elisha
Date: Thursday 16th October 2010

Elisha tells a story about making a huge sandcastle at the beach. They all talk about tasting salty seawater.

All of the children choose a puzzle each. Paul and Sara talk to each other. Elisha talks to Claire.

fuzzy felt

jigsaws

FI FI

AI M F

Elisha seems to be talking to both Sara and Holly in equal measure now. They decide to make a big seaside scene.

fuzzy felt

FI FI

6 1

5 2

4 3

A M F

jigsaws

Children choose another puzzle. Paul and Sara continue to chat. Elisha carries on with her quietly.

M FI FI

A M F FI

fuzzy felt

jigsaws

The girls talk about what they are making with the felt. Elisha mainly talks with Holly but sometimes to Sara They help each other to find the shapes they need. Paul finishes his puzzle and asks Claire if she'll play shop with him. They move to the role play area.

Holly comes to join the group. Elisha asks her if she'd like to do a puzzle. She says she's done them all and suggests fuzzy felt instead.

Observation schedules

More systematic forms of observation include the use of time sampling, event sampling and behavioural checklists. Using the *time sampling* technique, the observer notes down what a child does at specified intervals across a given time period. Time sampling can involve the simple narration of all action and speech but at given times (akin to a timed version of a running record), or it can specifically focus on recording particular behaviours in order to determine frequency patterns. Time period and behaviour can be broad, for example, noting the play type a child is engaged in at hour-long intervals throughout a 5-hour day. Alternatively, time period and behaviour can be specific, for example, recording social interaction across a 15-minute period at 1-minute intervals. (See Example 5 for time sampling.)

Example 5: Time sampling

Date: Monday 19th September 2010
Observer: Joyce
Aim: To note which areas of the club are being used by children each evening (3.30–5.30pm) at fifteen minute intervals

Time	Area				
	Sand	Art	Dress up	Carpet	Tables
3.30		✓✓	✓✓✓✓	✓✓✓✓	✓✓
3.45			✓✓✓✓	✓✓✓✓✓✓	✓✓✓✓
4.00	✓	✓✓	✓✓✓	✓✓✓	✓✓✓✓✓
4.15		✓✓	✓✓✓✓✓	✓✓✓✓✓	✓✓
4.30			✓✓✓✓	✓✓✓✓✓✓	✓✓✓✓
4.45	✓✓	✓	✓✓✓	✓✓✓	✓✓✓✓✓
5.00			✓✓✓✓	✓✓✓✓✓✓	✓✓✓✓
5.15			✓✓✓✓	✓✓✓✓✓✓	✓✓✓✓
5.30	✓✓	✓✓	✓✓✓✓	✓✓✓✓	✓✓
total	5	9	36	44	32

Notes:
The sand, water and art areas were used infrequently tonight and were used by the same few children each time (Maya, Ben, Ian and Therese). There seemed to be quite a lot of squabbling in the dress up area. Monitor this.

Event sampling is where the professional has identified a particular behaviour of interest and wishes to consider patterns of its occurrence. Once the behaviour has been identified, the professional makes notes whenever this behaviour occurs. Detail might include how long the behaviour persisted, along with details about context such as who else was present, where the behaviour occurred, what preceded the behaviour or how the behaviour ended. (See Example 6 for event sampling.)

Example 6: Event sampling

Date: Monday 26th & Tuesday 27th September 2010
Observer: Joyce
Aim: Squabbling observed in the dressing up area. Note the time, length of squabble, players involved along with details of the event. Also note if adult intervention required (AI)

Episode	Time	Duration	Who	Details	AI
1	3.45	3mins	Jo & Tom	Both wanted to have a turn at being a lion with the large yellow fur fabric	✓
2	4.00	1min	Paula & Di	Each wanted the same hat, they finally found another and had one each	
3	4.35	3mins	Elin & Sue	Each wanted a turn with the large netting to catch the lion in a trap	✓
4	5.00	1min	Bob & Tim	Bob said Tim had snatched something. Tim said didn't mean to snatch. Resolved quickly	
5	5.10	2mins	Finn & Jo	Both children wanted the large yellow fur	✓

Notes:
There didn't appear to be any pattern in the squabbling according to who was involved nor any gender difference. The children used the materials in lots of lovely ways, for example pretending to be different animals, to be a vet, a nurse or to make animal beds. Children generally resolved conflicts themselves except where large fabrics were involved, there were few of these available and the children liked to wrap themselves up in them or use them to make traps. These squabbles tended to go on for longer and adult intervention was often sought.

Using approaches cumulatively to develop an informative profile

It can also be useful to combine different types of observational records to inform our practice and to deepen our knowledge about a child's behaviour and development.

Elisha's change in sleep behaviour

From the diary entry in Example 1 above, we can see that Elisha's mum talked to the nursery manager because she was concerned about a change in her child's sleeping behaviour. The keyworkers thought that Elisha had been quieter than usual because her playmate Ellie was on holiday. They decided to monitor the situation and encourage her to play with others in the group. The activity clock is a record of their observation. Naomi found that, initially, Elisha only talked to the keyworker when she was doing her puzzle and not to the other children, Sara and Paul. The arrival of Holly, however, seemed to change the dynamic of the group, and during fuzzy felt play, Elisha talked with Holly and increasingly also with Sara. Naomi and Claire made an entry into Elisha's diary about the event and continued to encourage and monitor her social play. Elisha's mother said Elisha and Holly went to the same toddler group for a few weeks and perhaps she remembered her. After a day or so, she said Elisha seemed more like herself and that her usual sleep pattern had returned.

Molly and messy play

Joyce observed Molly's behaviour over several days using a tracking diagram, and found that she didn't take part in any art and craft activities. They decided to invite Molly to take part in a cutting and sticking activity, and made a running record of the session. Molly seemed to lack confidence in using the scissors, and the team decided to monitor this and also observe her fine motor skills in other types of play. In addition, however, Joyce also used time sampling to observe how children were using the various activities in the after-school club every evening. She found that few children were using the art and craft materials, and nor were they using the water and sand. Joyce asked the play team to talk to the children about what they liked and didn't like to do at club. Over the next few days the team reported that the children said they liked the messy play area but didn't use it much because there were no overalls and they were worried about getting their uniforms dirty. Old shirts were collected and used as aprons. A second time sample showed this area of the club was then used more frequently.

Squabbling in the dress-up area

Joyce originally time-sampled the children's activities at 15-minute intervals to find out how each activity was being used by children at the after-school club each day. As well as finding out that the messy play area was not used very often, Joyce noted that there seemed to be quite a lot of squabbling in the dress-up area compared to other activities. Event sampling behaviour in the dress-up area helped her to make sense of what was going on. Joyce had resisted pre-made dress-up costumes in favour of pieces of fabric in different colours and textures that could be used in a variety of ways. She observed that these were being used creatively, as she'd hoped, and that the children often negotiated how to take turns with the different items quite effectively. The most sustained squabbles related to sharing the very large pieces of fabric of which there were very few. It was felt that negotiating turns was an important skill, but that a few additional large pieces of fabric would be beneficial.

Supplementing your observational data

To be sure that we are considering children's development in social and cultural context, it is important that we use as many sources of information as possible. This might include supplementing narrative records, diary entries and observations with artefacts or photographs. Developing a contextual narrative using different types of evidence and artefacts is central to the socio-cultural 'learning stories' approach to documenting children's development in early education (Carr, 2001). Sometimes children will want to take home what they have made, they may want to dismantle it or even throw it away. This does not mean that a record cannot be made and, with the child's consent, taking a photograph is often well received, particularly if the child can also have a copy.

Previously, this type of documentation has been financially constrained owing to the high costs of instant film (e.g. Polaroid). With increasingly well-priced and high-quality digital cameras, however, photographic records are now far more accessible. Keep in mind, however, the caution we have already raised about product-based interpretation error.

If you feel inclined to make a judgement based on the product of the child's play then feel confident in talking to them about what they have done or made to find out more. If Andrew's teacher had have asked him about why he painted the black pictures, he might have told him straight away that it was because no other paint pots were left! Give the child a leading role in the discussion, however, and reflect on any bias that could have the potential to permeate your conversation.

We have talked about the value of practitioner diary entries, but it is also worth noting the usefulness of working with children to develop their own diaries or scrap books. This is a well-used technique in social work and play therapy, with a view to encouraging children to engage in discussion about difficult life events, to make sense of the past and present, or to create positive memories (Carroll, 1998). We can also learn a great deal about children's lives by valuing our everyday conversations with them and developing good professional relationships with their families.

Developing and maintaining professional relationships both within and across professional contexts is also important. In the increasingly integrated world of children's services it is not uncommon to have groups of professionals meeting together to share case history material in order to develop interventions, care or services packages

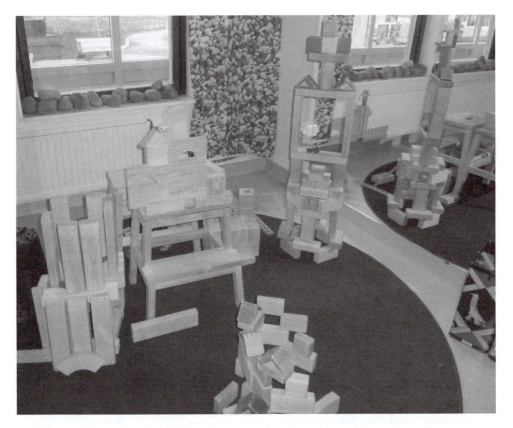

Children will often welcome you taking a photograph of their creations, especially where, for practical reasons, they have to be dismantled at some point. Many practitioners have a camera available for children to use themselves. In this photograph, also note the effective use of a mirrored wall, offering children an alternative visual perspective on both themselves and their creations

that best suit the needs of individual children and their families. It goes without saying, however, that discussion of case material occurs within the professional bounds of confidentiality. We must also remember that all of our observation or diary notes must be stored securely according to the Data Protection Act (1998).

Observing children at play

By observing children at play, we are able to consider their developing play skills as well as the developmental skills they are exhibiting as they play. In Chapter 2 we talked about how children's play progressed from that which is sensory and solitary in nature to that which involves symbolism and pretence, and then more complex cooperative games with rules. Movement through the play types both reflects and depends upon the development of skills and abilities across domains. Understanding this relationship means that we are able to provide experiences that promote a broad repertoire of play behaviour. It also means we are able to make more accurate judgements about play behaviour that deviates from that which we might ordinarily expect to observe. When observing and assessing children's play behaviour we might consider the presence of key play skills, sociability, the type of play exhibited or how engaged a child is with their play activity.

In Chapters 2 and 5 we discussed how play provided multiple opportunities for the development of physical, social and emotional, cognitive and language skills. When engaged in play, children often exhibit their highest levels of functioning and, as such, it provides a very positive measure of their development. When assessing children's health and development through play, you might consider the presence of key developmental milestones (e.g. in relation to language and communication or fine and gross motor control). Notwithstanding our caution regarding interpretation error, recurrent themes within a child's play might also be considered (e.g. if concerned about emotional health).

Useful measures to inform your assessment of play

- The Leuven Involvement Scale for Young Children (LIS-YC) is a tool for measuring children's engagement and wellbeing. It is simple to administer in a play-based context, and scores are easy to calculate and interpret.
- The Penn Interactive Peer Play Scale (PIPPS) is a behaviour observation schedule for measuring the sociability of play. It focuses on three areas: play interaction; play disruption; and play disconnection.
- The Developmental Play Assessment (DPA) tracks children's play behaviour across 15 levels. It provides an indication of the child's current play level and allows practitioners to design developmentally appropriate play-based interventions or activities based on sequential norms.
- The Play Skills Self Report Questionnaire (PSSRQ) is a useful tool, which asks children aged 5–10 years to reflect on their play skills, play activities and relationships during play. There is also a section for parental completion. It provides a useful overview of play behaviour upon which practice or interventions may be based.
- The Play Assessment for Group Settings measure (PAGS) is designed to evaluate children's play behaviour within social contexts. It is based on providing scores of between 1 (hardly ever) to 4 (nearly always) in response to a series of statements relating to a free child's play. The scale usefully includes a section on playful attitude.
- The Play Observation Scale (POS) is a system for recording basic play types and sociability. It is based on Piaget and Parten's theories of social and cognitive development in play.
- The Westby Play Scale (WPS) provides a useful developmental approach to assessing the progress of children's play from 18 months through to 5 years. It considers the props used in play, its thematic content, organisational elements, symbolism and language use.

Useful measures to inform your developmental assessment

- The Denver Developmental Screening Test (DDST) is widely used across children's services for the early identification of additional assessment requirements. The scale tracks the emergence of key developmental competencies across domains, from birth to 6 years. Most children's service teams will have a copy of this test.
- The Communication and Symbolic Behaviour Scale (CSBS) is a developmental profiling tool that can provide an early indication of the need for specialist speech and language assessment.
- The Behavioural and Emotional Rating Scale (BERS) is a 52-item scale, which evaluates the strengths of children aged 6–19 years in five areas: interpersonal strength; family involvement; intrapersonal strength; school functioning; and affective strength.
- The Rosenberg Self Esteem Scale is a short self-report measure, which contains 10 statements about the self that are answered on a four-point scale, from strongly agree to strongly disagree. Some items are reverse-scored. The higher the score, the higher the level of esteem.
- The Strengths and Difficulties Questionnaire (SDQ) is a brief emotional and behavioural assessment that can be completed in 5 minutes by parents or children's service professionals for children aged 4 to 16 years. There is a self-report version for 11–16-year-olds and a slightly modified version for practitioners working with children aged 3 years.

Now that you have read the chapter

- What are your current observation and assessment strategies? Are there any changes you might like to make or any new methods you could perhaps introduce?
- Go back through some of your previous observations. Are there any times when you might have been susceptible to interpretation error or professional bias?
- Do you feel confident enough in your knowledge of child development and developmental progression in play to make informed professional judgements about whether behaviour could be regarded as typical or atypical?
- Do you find any particular elements of observation challenging? Identify your strengths and weaknesses, and set yourself some professional development targets.

Useful further reading

Brassard, M. & Boehm, A. (2008) *Preschool Assessment: Principles and Practice* (London: Guildford Press).
This is a substantial book and would enrich the library of any children's service team. It is a useful reference text covering key elements of good assessment practice. It provides a critical review of an extensive range of assessments for young children across all developmental domains. Despite its title it includes reference to measures designed for children beyond pre-school age.

Gitlin-Weiner, K., Sandgrund, A. & Schaefer, C. (2002) *Play Diagnosis and Assessment* (London: John Wiley).
This is an invaluable resource for children's service professionals. It is a hardcover text and at more than £100 it is expensive, although second-hand copies can sometimes be picked up for less than half this price. It contains comprehensive details of scales and measures for assessment through play across domains.

8 Professional practice issues

Aims of the chapter

- To identify and discuss certain issues concerned with play practice.
- To discuss how these issues impact on the different play practices.
- To identify how taking children's perspectives of play might alleviate some of these issues.
- To identify how practitioners can share practice regarding these issues.

Introduction

Certain issues arise again and again when attempting to implement play, regardless of type of play practice. There is variation in how these issues affect play practice, depending upon the setting practitioners work in and the age of children practitioners work with. This chapter will discuss the following issues that impact on play practice:

- health and safety
- risk taking
- ethical practice
- boundary setting
- working with parents
- referral and safeguarding.

This chapter will identify generic aspects of each issue and well as specific ones related to each play practice. It will demonstrate how utilising children's perspectives of play might help in addressing some aspects of each issue and enable different play practitioners to share their understanding of each type of practice.

Health and safety

Perceptions of children's safety are heavily influenced by the media (Else, 2009). Parents are increasingly afraid to let their children out to play, and consequently children have reduced opportunities for free play. Research suggests that owing to parental fears up to one in three children do not play out on the street (Play England, 2010). It is further suggested that this curtailing of children's free play is contributing to a rise in mental health issues in children and young people (Mental Health Foundation, 1999, cited in Play England, 2010).

These fears have also affected children's play in school playgrounds, with children being banned from playing traditional games such as conkers. In recent years legislation concerned with safety has also impacted on outside play areas, with the height of climbing equipment being reduced, resulting in reduced opportunities for children to learn and develop.

These concerns and restrictions regarding children's safety while playing affect not only educational play practice, but also recreational play practice. Children have reduced space to play and reduced freedom and choice in their play, affecting their physical, emotional and social development (Palmer, 2006).

In order to ensure children's emotional safety and security, limit setting is an integral part of therapeutic play practice (West, 1996). Therapeutic play practitioners do not set many limits, but enough to secure children's physical safety while in the play room and their emotional security while playing. These limits are clearly communicated and reinforced as necessary with children. This also has the added advantage of ensuring adult wellbeing.

Playfulness and wellbeing would appear to be linked (Burdette & Whitaker, 2005; Gleave & Cole-Hamilton, 2012). Research suggests that utilising children's perceptions of play and creating situations where children feel playful would appear to be beneficial for children's overall wellbeing. A recent study (Howard & McInnes, 2012) has shown that manipulating children's perceptions of play to create playful and formal practice conditions results in children having a greater sense of wellbeing as measured using the Leuven Involvement Scale (Laevers, 2008; Laevers, Vandenbussche, Kog & Depondt, 1994).

Overall, it would appear that play practitioners can share practice in this area by drawing on therapeutic play practice and setting limits that ensure safety for children, and all practitioners can utilise children's perceptions of play to ensure children's wellbeing.

Risk taking

The concerns regarding health and safety outlined above also overlap with concerns regarding risk taking, for, as Gill (2007) notes, we live in an increasingly risk-averse society. Despite this, risk taking has been shown to be beneficial to all aspects of children's development (Gleave, 2008). As Waters and Begley (2007) state, taking physical risks in play enables children to take emotional, social and intellectual risks

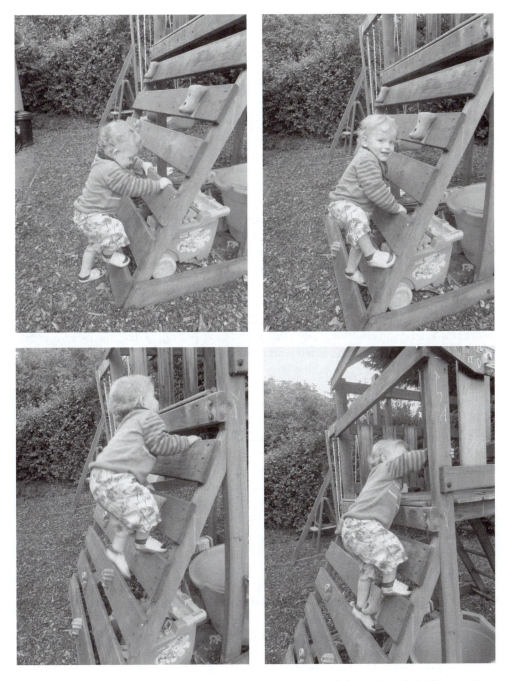

Not long after he was able to walk, this little one enjoyed the risk and challenge of getting to the top of the climbing frame in their play, thereby furthering these aspects of development. Additionally, children actually enjoy engaging in risky play, especially when connected with speed and heights, and actively seek out play experiences that include these elements (Sandseter, 2007; Stephenson, 2003).

However, although children enjoy risk taking, this viewpoint is not shared by parents and some play practitioners. Parents believe that children are exposed to more risks now than they used to be, and spend more time looking after them and supervising their play (Valentine, 2004). This fear of risk taking has also spread to children's play in schools and recreational play spaces (Gleave, 2008).

Recreational play practitioners recognise the need for children to engage in risky play, and Hughes (2001) discusses the benefits of deep play in recreational play practice, which is a type of play that brings children into contact with risk. However, educational play practitioners tend to be more reluctant to let children engage in risky play, and this is often not allowed in educational play spaces (Tovey, 2010). On the other hand, taking children to Forest Schools is acceptable, and there is recognition that children encounter risks in this environment and that it is beneficial to them (Tovey, 2007).

Overall, all play practitioners can learn from one another regarding risk taking and play. As recreational play practitioners already do, all play practitioners need to regard children as risk takers. Within therapeutic play practice risk taking by children is going to occur in relation to emotional risk taking, and limit setting, as described above, is put in to place to ensure children's safety and security. Within recreational and educational play practice, initially the risk taking is more likely to be physical risk taking, although this might lead into emotional risk taking.

Play practitioners need to provide an environment that supports children in engaging in physical risky play while setting limits to ensure safety-risk management (Gleave, 2008). As well as managing risk, play practitioners need to manage both their own and parents' anxiety concerning risk (Tovey, 2010). Sharing play practice with other practitioners is a good method by which to manage their own anxiety. Feeling secure about their practice and talking with parents about the value of risky play will go some way to alleviating parental anxiety.

Ethical practice

Ethical practice can be discussed in relation to working with children and in relation to research with children, both of which apply to play practitioners. Underpinning both of these aspects is that ethical practice should be founded on the fact that children have the right to a voice, in terms of saying what happens to them in relation to adult decision-making that affects them and to have their opinions taken into account as articulated in Article 12 of the United Nations Convention on the Rights of the Child (UNICEF, 2009). This directly affects their play as children need to have a say in their play and to make decisions about their play opportunities. Children need to be given a voice in relation to the resources they play with, the environment that is set up for them and the activities that are provided for them. In this way they can be in control of their play, which, as previously stated, is a component in children feeling playful.

In terms of feeling playful, another component related to control is having choice. Previous research has demonstrated that when children have choice about the activity or within the activity they feel more playful and performance is enhanced (McInnes, Howard, Miles & Crowley, 2009; Thomas, Howard & Miles, 2006). Having choice is a fundamental principle underpinning both recreational and therapeutic play practice, but, as discussed previously, educational play practice is not underpinned by such clear principles. Therefore, children being in control and having choice is less embedded in educational play practice. However, one study has shown that when educational practitioners have a clear understanding of play, they are more likely to afford children choice and control in their play (McInnes, Howard, Miles & Crowley, 2011).

Confidentiality and consent are important ethical aspects that apply to both practice and research. In therapeutic play practice children are respected, and what occurs in the playroom remains between therapist and child. In addition, it is important to gain consent from the child's legal guardian before commencing therapy (Landreth, 2012).

When conducting research with children, different play practitioners will have different ethical guidelines to follow. Therapeutic play practitioners may adhere to guidelines laid down by the British Association of Play Therapists (BAPT) or the British Psychological Society (BPS). Educational play practitioners will follow guidelines provided by the British Educational Research Association (BERA). These guidelines will include consent for children to participate in research. Informed consent, whereby legal guardians fully understand the nature of the research to be conducted, must be sought. In addition, consent should also be sought from the children, although this might not encompass fully informed consent, depending on the age of the children. Children should be asked if they would like to participate, and always be given the right to withdraw from the research process at any time.

In terms of giving consent and confidentiality, there might be times when breaking the confidence given is necessary. In cases where what is said during play practice or research gives cause for concern in terms of the health, welfare or safety of the child, then further action might need to be taken (Alderson & Morrow, 2004). The child will need to be informed that, from the information given, there are worries about their health, welfare or safety and that to protect them other people will need to be told. The matter then needs to be reported to the person responsible for child protection, and other professionals might need to be informed who will be able to act on behalf of the child.

The methodologies used for conducting research with children should always be appropriate. These may range from observing children and talking with children to using more experimental methodologies, such as the AASP discussed in Chapter 4. Using audio and visual recording equipment with children is common across both practice and research. In practice recording children's work or their play is a frequent occurrence. It enables practitioners to reflect on their practice and on children and to make changes for the benefit of children. In research it is a frequently used methodology to listen to children's perspectives. However, this is fraught with dilemmas and raises many ethical questions in terms of confidentiality, anonymity and effects on participants (Robson, 2011).

Boundary setting

All play practitioners need to set boundaries or limits when working with children. These may be professional boundaries, practice boundaries and/or emotional boundaries. Having boundaries creates a safe and acknowledged framework within which practitioners can work. Knowing and respecting each other's professional boundaries will enable practitioners to know when, and how, to refer to other agencies. This will ensure that children and their families get appropriate and correct advice and help when needed. It should also ensure that information is shared between practitioners, and support and advance multi-agency working.

Setting boundaries is beneficial for children too. It provides children with knowledge regarding what is and is not acceptable. It also provides children with security and consistency, which is useful for building relationships. However, it is important to recognise that setting boundaries does not preclude children from having a sense of freedom and control or from approaching tasks playfully. Having boundaries provides children with a safe context in which they can exercise freedom and control, and take a playful attitude and approach to activities.

Setting practice boundaries is common across all play practitioners. Educational play practitioners set classroom rules that agree limits for children's play and behaviour. At times this might appear to cut across children's play or play opportunities, but is deemed necessary to ensure appropriate and safe behaviour within a setting. Recreational play practitioners follow the playwork principles, which foreground children's choice within play. However, play practitioners conduct risk assessments to ensure children's safety, and in this way may set some limits for their play.

Therapeutic limit or boundary setting is an integral part of therapeutic play practice (Landreth, 2012). This is limit setting, which ensures safe practice and security for the child, and facilitates psychological growth. Some of the limits that might be set have been discussed above under health and safety. Further limits might be set to ensure a professional and socially acceptable relationship between therapist and child. An example is setting limits on overtly sexual behaviour by children by stating that this type of inappropriate behaviour is unacceptable.

There are recognised stages to limit setting within therapeutic play practice. Firstly, the wishes and feelings underlying the unacceptable behaviour are recognised and acknowledged. This ensures that while the behaviour may be unacceptable the feelings are real and accepted. For example, if a child throws a toy at the therapist the therapist would recognise and acknowledge the feeling behind the behaviour: 'you are angry with me'. Secondly, the limits of the unacceptable behaviour are verbalised clearly: 'you cannot throw the brick at me'. Thirdly, more acceptable behaviours are provided: 'you can throw the brick in the box' (for a more detailed description of limit setting within therapeutic practice, see Landreth, 2012, pp. 271–5).

Emotional boundary setting should be considered by all play practitioners to protect them from becoming too involved in children's lives or using play to meet their own needs. Discussing practice and children's play with other practitioners through daily or weekly team meetings is one way of ensuring that the emotional burden is shared and best practice is provided. Within therapeutic play practice, personal therapy or counselling is a professional requirement that ensures the emotional health of the practitioner and enables effective practice (West, 1996). This, together with the step-by-step limit setting described above, are practices that could be shared by all play practitioners in their play with children.

Working with parents

For most children, at least in Western cultures, play begins in the home (Smith, 2010). Parents are their children's first play partners, and it is playful interaction that forms the basis of the children's attachment (Pellegrini, 2009). Playful interactions that are meaningful and sensitive, with adults who are sensitive to the communicative cues provided through games such as pat-a-cake and peek-a-boo, provide children with a secure base. It also provides them with an understanding of, and expectations for, future playful behaviour.

However, despite these early shared play behaviours, parents tend to have different perceptions of play compared to play professionals. While appearing positive about play, as highlighted above, parents are fearful about their children playing outside and of engaging in risky play behaviours. In addition, pressure from within the education system leads parents into valuing learning outcomes and believing that this might not be achievable through play (Fung & Cheng, 2012; Palmer, 2006).

Therefore, all play practitioners need to work with parents to, first of all, communicate the value of play for their children so that parents will understand the necessity of children engaging in play. For recreational play practitioners this aspect of their practice is underpinned by the principle that states that practitioners should act as advocates for children's play. Although not directly concerned with enabling parents to understand the value of play, it may be reinterpreted in this way as it involves practitioners questioning adult agendas around play and standing up for children's right to play (Conway, 2008).

Educational play practitioners frequently engage in conversation with parents concerning what children are learning through play. They may also hold open evenings and discovery mornings with practical hands-on activities that parents can engage in with their children in order to help parents understand the value of play in an educational context (Smidt, 2011). Moyles (1989) identifies five aspects of play that usually help parents to understand play better. These aspects are concerned with motivation; the freedom to make mistakes; the ability to work through problems; to understand one's own learning; and the fact that even adults engage in recreation and learn through play.

As stated above, therapeutic play practitioners need to gain consent from the child's legal guardian, who is usually the parent, before commencing therapy. Therapeutic play practice is clearly explained to the parent so that they understand what their child is going to be engaging with through this play practice. In addition, there are some types of therapeutic play practice that directly involve the parent, such as filial play therapy in which the parent is helped to become a therapist to their child (Van Fleet, 2005). Outcome studies have shown this particular play therapy intervention to be effective (Bratton, Ray, Rhine & Jones, 2005).

Once the value of play is explained to parents they may take a more favourable stance toward play, and enable their children to engage in more playful opportunities. It is also suggested that children's perceptions of play are explained to parents and the value of practitioners talking with them highlighted. It may also be useful for parents to directly talk with children about their play, not necessarily about the detail of what they do when they play, but about what they think play is and what they value during play.

Referral and safeguarding

Hill, Head, Lockyer, Reid and Taylor (2012) summarise evidence that demonstrates the benefits of inter-agency working. Among these are increased knowledge sharing and reduced duplication, and a more holistic approach to understanding the needs of children and families. However, they also identify the challenges of such an approach, in particular the need for effective communication between agencies and the availability of resources to facilitate such communication, a shared and consistent language and knowledge base and, importantly, a transparent and standardised framework for assessment, recording and referral.

To ensure that professionals across children's services take a consistent approach in working together to support the health and wellbeing of all children at a national level, a continuum of needs has been identified, which is used as a framework for the identification of and provision for additional needs. Frameworks are based on the five key outcomes of Every Child Matters (DfES, 2004b) and the Children Act (DfES,

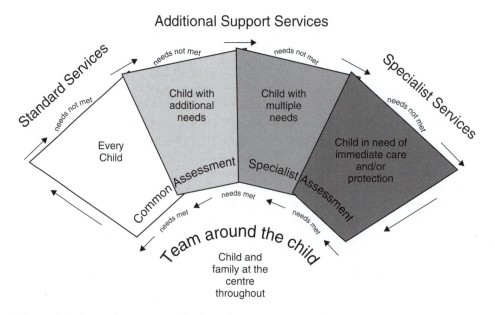

Figure 8.1 A continuum model of needs assessment and service provision

2004a). These include: being healthy; staying safe; enjoying and achieving; making a positive contribution to society; and achieving economic wellbeing. Many authorities adopt a continuum model to guide practitioners in their assessments of children's needs such as that depicted in Figure 8.1.

The frameworks recognise that the majority of children will have needs that can be met by parents or primary caregivers and standard health, educational or social care services but also that other children will require support from specialist services or multiple agencies working together. The Bolton Framework for Action (Bolton Safeguarding Board, 2007) is one such example of this type of approach. Levels of need and possible indicators of need, along with suggested professional response, are presented in Table 8.1.

Table 8.1 The Framework for Action (Bolton Safeguarding Board, 2007)

Level of need	Possible indicators and action
Every child Children whose needs across the five key outcomes are being addressed	• The child is physically and mentally healthy • The child is safe from physical and emotional harm • They are achieving developmental and educational milestones • They engage positively with society • The child is confident and well supported **Action:** None required, needs are being addressed via current services and parent/carer provision
Level 1 Children with additional needs whose health and development may be affected	• Children with mental or physical health difficulties • Children with isolated, unsupported carer(s) • Children in families where there is poor hygiene • Children identified by schools as requiring additional educational support, including behavioural, emotional and social difficulties • Children starting to have unauthorised absences from school • Children who have started involvement in criminal activities • Children involved in contact/residence disputes • Children of parents involved in substance misuse • Children experimenting with drugs/substances • Children of parents where there has been some domestic abuse • Children who have episodes of missing from home • Families with a high number of children or more than two under 5 • Young carers • Children experiencing bullying • Young people disengaged from education, training or employment post-16

Table 8.1 Continued

Level of need	Possible indicators and action
	• Carers under stress • Carers not accessing appropriate services • Carers struggling to manage children's behaviour • Carers with mental, physical difficulties and or learning difficulties **Action:** The needs of the child are assessed within the worker's own agency. This may involve use of a standard assessment proforma within the worker's context or use of a Common Assessment Framework (CAF). If circumstances are not improved after current resources have been accessed/ maximised then the worker should consider referral to additional specialist assessment
Level 2 Children with additional needs whose health and development is at increased risk of being affected	• Children with increasing behavioural, emotional or social difficulties • Children regularly absent from school • Homeless children/young people • Children with chronic ill health or terminal illness • Children previously on the Child Protection Register • Children returning to their parents having been looked after by the local authority • Children in families where there are emerging patterns of domestic abuse • Children/young people with substance dependency • Children who are regularly missing from home • Children who consistently miss medical appointments and/or treatment • Children consistently not seen by one or more agencies • Carers unable to meet their children's basic needs as a result of extreme poverty • Carers who have substance misuse dependency which impacts on their ability to meet their children's needs • Carers with chronic ill health or terminal illness • Carers with moderate learning difficulties or physical disabilities • Carers experiencing mental health difficulties **Action:** The child may have multiple needs requiring service co-ordination or may require support services not currently available through the worker's own agency. An action meeting will be organised and a professional will be dedicated to leading an action plan.

Table 8.1 Continued

Level of need	Possible indicators and action
Level 3 Children who have complex needs whose health and development is being affected	• Children with significant behavioural, emotional or social difficulties • Children in households where parents/carers have multiple problems • Children with families experiencing a crisis likely to result in a breakdown of care arrangements • Children in families where there has been one significant episode of domestic abuse or continuing incidents • Children/young people with chaotic and or poly substance misuse • Carers who do not consistently meet the basic needs of their children • Carers with chaotic and or poly substance misuse • Carers with significant learning difficulties or physical disabilities • Carers with significant mental health difficulties **Action:** Specialist assessment is undertaken by children's services.
Level 4 Children at risk of or suffering significant harm in need of protection or substitute care	• Children who are at risk of/are suffering abuse or neglect including unborn children • Children with unexplained injuries, suspicious injuries or where there is an inconsistent explanation of the injury • Children who have non-organic faltering growth • Unaccompanied asylum-seeking children • Privately fostered children and young people • Children whose behaviour is sufficiently extreme to place them at risk of removal from home, e.g. risky behaviour, dangerous behaviour, involvement in sexual exploitation • Children who disappear or are missing from home regularly or for long periods • Children subject to proceedings initiated by the local authority • Unborn babies where previous child protection concerns have been identified • Carers unable to address their children's needs whether for physical, intellectual, emotional or social reasons **Action:** Requires immediate referral to the appropriate children's service team.

Adapted from the Framework for Action, Bolton Safeguarding Board (2007, Section A1)

Conclusion

In this chapter a variety of practice issues common across all play practices have been discussed: health and safety, risk taking, ethical practice, setting boundaries, working with parents and referrals and safeguarding. However, how these issues affect the different play practices varies. It is hoped that by discussing these differences all play practitioners can gain insight and understanding into each other's practice and learn new ways of dealing with these issues. Ultimately, by sharing practice this should enable children to have more play opportunities that enable them to take risks, thereby benefiting their health and wellbeing. Valuing and working with parents, setting safe and appropriate boundaries and engaging in ethical practice and research will also increase and improve play opportunities for children as well as increasing our knowledge about children's play.

Now that you have read the chapter

- Are you aware of the referral and safeguarding process in your setting? Find the policy, read and reflect.
- Are you happy that you are working effectively with the parents of the children in your setting? Reflect on your current practice. Is there scope for improvement?
- Reflect on the boundaries and rules you set for children when they play. Are these boundaries and rules always necessary and always for the child's benefit?
- Does your setting allow children to take risks? How do perceptions of risk and safety differ among colleagues in your setting?

Useful further reading

There is no one key text that addresses all the above issues, therefore a selection of texts is suggested for different issues.

Else, P. (2009). *The Value of Play*. London: Continuum. *See Chapter 2 for health and safety, and risk taking.*

Harcourt, D., Perry, B. & Waller, T. (2011). *Researching Young Children's Perspectives*. London: Routledge, *for ethical practice.*

Hill, M., Head, G., Lockyer, A., Reid, B. & Taylor, R. (2012) *Children's Services: Working Together*. London: Pearson, *for working together, referrals and safeguarding.*

Landreth, G. L. (2012). *Play Therapy: The Art of the Relationship*, 3rd edn. New York: Routledge. *See Chapter 11 for setting boundaries.*

Moyles, J. (1989). *Just Playing?* Buckingham: Open University Press. *See Chapter 9 for working with parents.*

Conclusion

Throughout the book we have tried to forefront that autonomy and control and fundamental to children's play. Play is important in the 'here and now', and the qualities associated with the 'here and now' experience are effectively what renders play so inherently valuable for development across domains in the longer term. We propose that the benefits associated with play across contexts are closely related to its unique capacity to promote and maintain a positive sense of self and, as such, play acts as a resource enabling children to meet physical, intellectual and emotional challenges (see Introduction).

Conceptualising play from children's perspectives is of central importance to all play professionals. The benefits associated with children taking a playful approach to their activities cannot be differentiated across contexts and, as such, it is vital that all professionals working with play appreciate its powerful developmental and therapeutic potential. Understanding these characteristics provides an opportunity for professionals to offer authentic play experiences whether these are directed toward recreational, health, educational or therapeutic outcomes.

In recent years reports have highlighted concerns about children's emotional wellbeing, especially in the UK. UNICEF noted high levels of unhappiness among children in the UK, with only children from the US faring worse (UNICEF, 2009). Good emotional wellbeing can protect children against a variety of problems in the future, including: emotional and behavioural problems, violence and crime, and teenage pregnancy (NICE, 2008). Recognition as to the importance of play for children's development across domains has resulted in initiatives designed to ensure access to appropriate play opportunities from a health, education and social care perspective right across the UK (Powell & Wellard, 2008). There is particular emphasis on early intervention, and school-based programmes such as SEAL (Social and Emotional Aspects of Learning) focus on building resiliency, confidence and esteem.

These play-based strategies are not only important for increasing awareness about emotional health and reducing the stigma children associate with receiving counselling or therapy (Cowie, 2012), but may also prevent some children from needing to access these higher-tier mental care services. Increased recognition as to the value of play for ensuring children's emotional health and development, however, must also be reflected

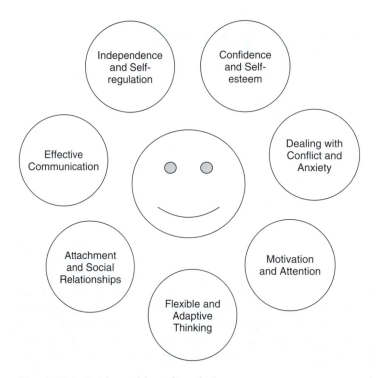

Figure C.1 Evidenced benefits of play

in the training opportunities made available for children's service professionals. Everyone working with children and young people would benefit from a shared understanding as to the developmental and therapeutic significance of play. This is particularly important given that relatively recent research indicates that only a minority (10–20 per cent) of children with mental health problems are referred for specialist support, the remainder having to deal with their difficulties as best they can with the support of those around them (Rutter, Kim-Cohen & Maughan, 2006).

Effective play practice relies on us being confident about the reasons why play is important for children's development, and developing a personal philosophy based on research evidence to guide our practice (Howard, 2010b). We propose that there are particular evidence-based features of play that suggest that play contributes to emotional wellbeing and that emotional wellbeing lays the foundation for all professional practice. Play makes a significant contribution to children's emotional health and subsequently enhances development across domains by supporting seven forms of development, as follows.

Attachment and other social relationships

Play contributes to the healthy development of early attachment bonds, for example, in games like 'peek-a-boo', gentle rocking to a soothing lullaby or touch-and-tickle games like 'round and round the garden'. These warm and trusting relationships provide the child with a secure base from which they develop the confidence to explore the world around them, and also play a vital role in the development of what Bowlby (1997) describes as the Internal Working Model (IWM). The IWM is an internal system that the child uses to shape their growing relationships with others. Play provides valuable opportunities for the development of these new relationships (Panksepp, 2007), and also, where attachments are insecure or have been broken, it can function to restore and rebuild confidence and trust. Positive play experiences can serve to remodel the IWM and contribute to many therapeutic techniques for children who have attachment difficulties.

Effective communication

Vygotsky (1978) argued that play was one of the first ways that children explore symbols, and through pretence they learn that one thing can stand for or symbolise another. In this sense, it makes an invaluable contribution to the development of future language ability. Play offers a wealth of opportunities for children to develop verbal and nonverbal communication skills. They learn about turn-taking, negotiation and behavioural adjustments according to context or company. Children may use play as a means of communicating their thoughts and feelings, and might play out difficult or painful experiences (McMahon, 2009). In a playful environment where children feel safe and in control of events, they may be more likely to talk about any issues that are worrying them (Li & Lopez, 2008) as well as talking about their lives in general. This contributes to the growth and development of existing and new relationships. Engaging with children as a play partner enables us to get to know them, and communicates to them that we value what they say and do. During play we are able to model actions and emotions, and because of the increased attention associated with activities children perceive to be play, these are more likely to be repeated.

Independence and self-regulation

An important element of children's development is their growing independence and ability to manage their behaviour and emotions. Even during early sensory play, babies learn about their physical self and that their actions impact on the environment and those around them. Gradually, as behaviour becomes more purposeful, cause and effect are recognised. Being able to manage and control our behaviour (to self-regulate) develops over time. As adults, many of our behaviours have become automatic and are done without needing to think. When we are faced with a problem or challenge, our thinking generally happens in our heads. Behavioural automaticity develops over time, as does the ability to silently think things through. In early childhood, self-regulation occurs externally, and children think out loud when faced with new or challenging situations. We can observe children talking through what they are doing in their play, and this often reflects their actions or a strategy they are using to deal with a problem.

The development of self-regulatory skills is vital to development across domains, and children use more self-regulatory language in activities they see as play rather than not play (Whitebread, 2010).

Confidence and self-esteem

Resilient children are those who have a balanced outlook on life and a positive sense of self (Masten & Coatsworth, 1998). When children are engaged in play they are provided with opportunities to develop confidence in their abilities as any goals are self-set. This reduces the impact of failure but still enables children to learn about their strengths and limitations. Children learn to master skills through play, and a sense of mastery and achievement contributes to the development of self-esteem and the ability to approach new challenges with confidence. Children show higher levels of involvement in activities they perceive as play. Involvement is based on flow states, and increased involvement in an activity is reported to indicate greater emotional wellbeing. Indicators of involvement include: deep concentration, strong motivation, satisfaction and positive energy (Laevers, 2008) These indicators overlap with those used in children's self reports of self-esteem and wellbeing (Fattore, Mason & Watson, 2007).

Strategies for dealing with conflict and anxiety

As previously discussed, play can be a useful medium for children to communicate their thoughts and feelings. The 'unreal' aspect of play, however, is particularly important. Sutton-Smith (2003) proposes that play enables us to experience primary emotions that could threaten to overwhelm us in our everyday life. It can provide distance, enabling children to cope with difficult emotions within the safety of their own play space, for example, through playing out a scenario with small world toys. Further distance can be created by the use of metaphor, for example, through stories, music or drama. Timberlake and Cutler (2001) propose that metaphor can transform complex issues into a language children can readily understand. Jennings (1999) proposes that dramatic distance paradoxically brings children closer to being able to deal with trauma and anxiety. Play provides a language by which children can encode, store, retrieve and make sense of their experiences. Play experiences offer opportunities to create positive memories that contribute to our life stories. While engaged in play, children can become desensitised to particular fears or phobias. Therapists may use focused play techniques to encourage children to access repressed or unresolved issues that may be stored in the unconscious mind. Play can act as a cue for remembering, enabling children to retrieve information more effectively (Schaefer, 2011). It is important to remember, however, that play can act as a cue to both positive and negative emotions. As research evidence increasingly alerts us to the importance of enabling autonomy and control in children's play, it also becomes increasingly possible that children may play out conflict or anxiety in their spontaneous play.

Flexible and adaptive thinking

Theories of play, which centralise the freedom, choice and control children have in play activities, emphasise its role in promoting flexible thinking skills. The ability to adapt and be flexible is a further characteristic of the resilient child (Masten, 2001). In play, children are able to make novel connections, express individuality and creativity, and develop their imaginations. Observing children at play, we are able to see progression in the way children think about objects they encounter, and the pattern of 'What is this?', 'What does this do?', 'What can I do with this?' and 'What could I do with this?' continues through the lifespan (Craft, 2005).

Motivation and attention

High levels of attention and motivation can be observed when children are at play, and as we saw in Chapter 3, they are less distracted in activities that afford them choice and control. Barsalou (2008) looks at the significance of embodied experience in the retrieval of memories. and the impact of this on a person's ability to respond to present circumstances. His theory of grounded cognition suggests that the more present and aware we are for an original experience, the better our recall will be. Attention and motivation are important elements in modelling and imitation (Bandura, 1973). There is a significant difference in the amount of time an adult can sustain a child's attention for in a directed task at 2 years of age compared with a child of 6 years (5 minutes compared with 50 minutes). What is noticeable, however is that children are able to concentrate for long periods in their self-directed play from a very early age. Several studies report children's increased level of motivation and enthusiasm during play. If children are in control over what they play, where, with whom and for how long, then their attention is more easily maintained.

References

Abbott, L. & Langston, A. (2005). *Birth to Three Matters: Supporting the Framework for Effective Practice.* Maidenhead: Open University Press.

Ahonen-Eerikäinen, H., Lamont, A. & Knox, R. (2008). Rehabilitation for children with cerebral palsy: Seeing through the looking glass – enhancing participation and restoring self-image through the virtual music instrument. *International Journal of Psychosocial Rehabilitation. 12(2):* 41–66.

Ainsworth, M., Blehar, M., Waters, E. & Wall, S. (1978). *Patterns of Attachment.* Hillsdale, NJ: Erlbaum.

Alderson, P. & Morrow, V. (2004). *Ethics, Social Research and Consulting with Children and Young People.* Barkingside: Barnardo's.

Alharbi, A. (2012). Exploring perceptions of play therapy and the utilisation of play therapy in Saudi Arabia. Unpublished Master's Thesis. Swansea University.

Anning, A. & Edwards, A. (2006). *Promoting Children's Learning from Birth to Five Years: Developing the New Early Years Professional.* Maidenhead: Open University Press.

Ariès, P. (1960). *Centuries of Childhood.* Harmondsworth: Penguin Books.

Axline, V. (1979). *Dibs In Search of Self: Personality Development in Play Therapy.* London: Penguin.

Axline, V. (1989). *Play Therapy.* Boston, MA: Houghton Mifflin.

Bandura, A. (1973). *Aggression in Social Learning Analysis.* Englewood Cliffs, NJ: Prentice Hall.

Barnett, L. A. (2007). The nature of playfulness in young adults. *Personality and Individual Differences, 43:* 949–958.

Barsalou, L. W. (2008). Grounded cognition. *Annual Review of Psychology, 59:* 617645.

Bennett, N., Wood, L. & Rogers, S. (1997). *Teaching Through Play.* Buckingham: Open University Press.

Bodrova, E. & Leong, D. J. (2007). *Tools of the Mind: The Vygotskian Approach to Early Childhood Education* (2nd edn). Upper Saddle River, NJ: Pearson/Merrill Prentice Hall.

Bolton Safeguarding Board. (2007). *Framework for Action: For all Children, Young People and Families.* Bolton: Bolton Safeguarding Board.

Bowlby, J. (1969). *Attachment and Loss,* vol. 1: *Attachment.* New York: Basic Books.

Bowlby, J. (1997). *Attachment and Loss,* vol. 2: *Separation, Anxiety and Anger.* London: Pimlico Books [originally published 1973].

Brassard, M. & Boehm, A. (2008). *Preschool Assessment: Principles and Practice.* London: Guildford Press.

Bratton, S. & Ray, D. (2000). What the research shows about play therapy. *International Journal of Play Therapy, 9(1)*: 47–88.

Bratton, S., Ray, D., Rhine, T. & Jones, L. (2005). The efficacy of play therapy with children: A meta-analytic review of treatment outcomes. *Professional Psychology: Research and Practice, 36(4)*: 376–390.

Broadhead, P. (2010). Cooperative play and learning from nursery to year 1. In P. Broadhead, J. Howard & E. Wood (Eds), *Play and Learning in the Early Years* (pp. 43–59). London: Sage.

Bronfenbrenner, U. (1979). *The Ecology of Human Development*. Cambridge, MA: Harvard University Press.

Bronson, M. R. & Bundy, A. C. (2001). A correlational study of a test of playfulness and a test of environmental supportiveness for play. *Occupational Therapy Journal of Research, 21(4)*: 241–259.

Brooker, L. (2001). Interviewing children. In G. MacNaughton, S. A. Rolfe & I. Siraj-Blatchford (Eds), *Doing Early Childhood Research: International Perspectives on Theory and Practices* (pp. 162–177). Buckingham: Open University Press.

Brown, F. (2003). *Playwork: Theory and Practice*. Buckingham: Open University Press.

Brown, F. (2008). The fundamentals of playwork. In F. Brown & C. Taylor (Eds), *Foundations of Playwork*. (pp. 7–13). Buckingham: Open University Press.

Bruce, T. (2011). Froebel today. In L. Miller & L. Pound (Eds), *Theories and Approaches to Learning in the Early Years* (pp. 55–70). London: Sage.

Bruner, J. S. (1972). Nature and uses of immaturity. *American Psychologist*, 687–708.

Bruner, J. S. (1974). *Toward a Theory of Instruction*. Cambridge, MA: Belknap Press.

Bukatko, D. & Daehler, M. W. (2011). *Child Development: A Thematic Approach*. Andover: Cengage Learning.

Bundy, A. C., Shia, S., Qi, L. & Miller, L. J. (2007). How does sensory processing dysfunction affect play? *American Journal of Occupational Therapy, 61*: 201–208.

Burdette, H. L. & Whitaker, R. C. (2005). Resurrecting free play in young children. *Archives of Pediatric & Adolescent Medicine, 159*: 46–50.

Burghardt, G. M. (2005). *The Genesis of Animal Play*. Cambridge, MA: MIT Press.

Burghardt, G. M. (2011). Defining and recognizing play. In A. D. Pellegrini (Ed.), *The Oxford Handbook of the Development of Play* (pp. 9–18). Oxford: Oxford University Press.

Bussey, K. & Bandura, A. (1999) Social cognitive theory or gender development and differentiation. *Psychological Review, 106(4)*: 676–713.

Carr, M. (2001). *Assessment in Early Childhood Settings: Learning Stories*. London: Sage.

Carroll, J. (1998) *Introduction to Therapeutic Play*. London: Blackwell Science.

Carruthers, E. & Worthington, M. (2005). Making sense of mathematical graphics: The development of understanding abstract symbolism. *European Early Childhood Education Research Journal, 13(1)*: 57–79.

Chapman, L. (2011). The importance of age and experience in the development of children's perceptions of play. Unpublished MSc Dissertation, University of Glamorgan.

Chapman, L. M. (2010). *Inclusivity*. Available from: www.equalitytraining.co.uk.

Children Act (1989) [online]. HMSO1989 (c.41). Available from: www.hmso.gov.uk.

Children Act (2004) [online]. HMSO2004 (c.31). Available from: www.hmso.gov.uk.

Cohen, D. (2006). *The Development of Play* (3rd edn). London: Routledge.

Conway, M. (2008). The playwork principles. In F. Brown & C. Taylor (Eds), *Foundations of Playwork* (pp. 119–123). Maidenhead: Open University Press.

Cowie, H. (2012). *From Birth to Sixteen: Children's Health, Social, Emotional and Linguistic Development*. London: Routledge.

Craft, A. (2005). *Creativity in Schools: Tensions and Dilemmas*. London: Routledge.

Crain, W. C. (2005). *Theories of Development: Concepts and Applications* (5th edn). Upper Saddle River, NJ: Pearson/Prentice Hall.

Csikszentmihalyi, M. (1979). The concept of flow. In B. Sutton-Smith (Ed.), *Play and Learning* (pp. 257–274). New York: Gardner Press Inc.

Csikszentmihalyi, M. (1988). The flow experience and human psychology. In M. Csikszentmihalyi & I. S. Csikszentmihalyi (Eds), *Optimal Experience: Psychological Studies of Flow in Consciousness* (pp. 15–35). Cambridge: Cambridge University Press.

Csikszentmihalyi, M. (1990). *Flow: The Psychology of Optimal Experience*. New York: HarperCollins Publishers.

Dahlberg, G., Moss, P. & Pence, A. (2007). *Beyond Quality in Early Childhood Education and Care*. London: Routledge.

Data Protection Act (1998). London: Stationery Office. Available at: www.legislation. gov.uk.

Davey, C. & Lundy, L. (2011). Towards greater recognition of the right to play: An analysis of Article 31 of the UNCRC. *Children and Society, 25(1)*: 3–14.

David, T., Goouch, K., Powell, S. & Abbott, L. (2003). *Birth to Three Matters: A Review of the Literature*. Nottingham: DfES Publications.

Davis-Berman, J. & Berman, D. (2008). *The Promise of Wilderness Therapy*. Boulder, CO: Association for Experiential Education.

DCSF (2007). *The Children's Plan: Building Brighter Futures*. Nottingham: DCSF Publications.

DCSF (2008). *Fair Play: A Commitment from the Children's Plan*. Nottingham: DCSF Publications.

Department of Health (2005). *National Service Framework for Children, Young People and Maternity Services*. Available from: www.dh.gov.uk

Deutsch, J., Borbely, M., Filler, J., Huhn, K. & Guarrera-Bowlby, P. (2008) Use of a low-cost, commercially available gaming console (Wii) for rehabilitation of an adolescent with cerebral palsy. *Physical Therapy, 88(10)*: 1196–1207.

Dewey, J. (1933). *How We Think*. Boston, MA: D. C. Heath and Company.

DfES (2004a). The Children Act [online]. HMSO2004 (c.31). Available from: www.hmso.gov.uk.

DfES (2004b). *Every Child Matters: Change for Children*. Nottingham: DfES Publications.

Disability Discrimination Act (DDA) (2005) [online]. HMSO2005 (c.13). Available from: www.hmso.gov.uk.

Doherty, J. (2009). Play for children with Special Needs. In A. Brock, S. Dobbs, P. Jarvis & Y. Olusga (Eds), *Perspectives on Play*. London: Pearson.

Doyle, J. (2006). Nature makes the best teacher and classroom. *Early Years Educator, 8(3)*: Forest School Supplement, ii–x.

Drummond, M. (1999). Another way of seeing: Perceptions of play in a Steiner kindergarten. In L. Abbott & H. Moylett (Eds), *Early Education Transformed* (pp. 48–60). London: Falmer Press.

Dunn, J. (1997). The impact of sensory processing abilities on the daily lives of young children and their families: A conceptual model. *Young Children 9(4)*: 23–35.

Dykas, M. & Cassidy, J. (2011). Attachment and the processing of social information across the life span: Theory and evidence. *Psychological Bulletin, 137(1)*: 19–46.

Dyspraxia Foundation (2012). *The Symptoms*. Accessed online at: www.dyspraxia foundation.org.uk.

Eisele, G. & Howard, J. (2012). Exploring the presence of characteristics associated with play within the ritual repetitive behavior of autistic children. *International Journal of Play, 1(2)*.

Eisert, D. & Lamorey, S. (1996). Play as a window on child development: The relationship between play and other developmental domains. *Early Education and Development, 7(3)*: 221–235.

Elias, C. & Berk, L. (2002). Self-regulation in young children: Is there a role for sociodramatic play? *Early Childhood Research Quarterly, 17*: 216–238.

Else, P. (2009). *The Value of Play*. London: Continuum.

Epstein, A., Schweinhart, L., DeBruin-Parecki, A. & Robin, K. (2004). *Preschool Assessment: A Guide to Developing a Balanced Approach*. National Institute for Early Education Research. Accessed online at: http://nieer.org/resources/policybriefs/7.pdf.

Epstein L., Roemmich, J., Robinson, J., Paluch, R., Winiewicz, D. Fuerch, J. & Robinson, T. (2007). A randomized trial of the effects of reducing television viewing and computer use on Body Mass Index in young children. *Paediatric Adolescent Medicine, 62(3)*: 239–245.

Erikson, E. H. (1963). *Childhood and Society* (2nd edn). New York: W. W. Norton.

Fagan, R. M. (1984). Play and behavioural flexibility. In P. K. Smith (Ed.), *Play in Animals and Humans* (pp. 159–173). Oxford: Blackwell.

Fattore, T., Mason, J. & Watson, E. (2007). Children's conceptualisation(s) of their well-being. *Social Indicators Research, 80*: 5–29.

Fawcett, M. (1996). *Learning Through Child Observation*. London: Jessica Kingsley Press.

Fawcett, M. (2000). Historical views of childhood. In M. Boushel, M. Fawcett & J. Selwyn (Eds), *Focus on Early Childhood: Principles and Realities* (pp. 7–20). Oxford: Blackwell Science Ltd.

Fearn, M. & Howard, J. (2011). Play as resource for children facing adversity: An exploration of indicative case studies. *Children & Society*, doi: 10.1111/j.1099-0860.2011.00357.

Fincher, W., Shaw, J. & Ramelet, A. S. (2012). The effectiveness of a standardised preoperative preparation in reducing child and parent anxiety: A single-blind randomised controlled trial. *Journal of Clinical Nursing, 21(7)*: 946–955.

Fisher-Thompson, D. (1993). Adult toy purchases for children: Factors affecting sex typed toy selection. *Journal of Applied Developmental Psychology, 14*: 385–406.

Fjortoft, I. (2004). Landscapes as playscape: The effects of natural environments on children's play and motor development. *Children Youth and Environments, 14(2)*: 21–44.

Fung, C. K. H. & Cheng, D. P. W. (2012). Consensus or dissensus? Stakeholders' views on the role of play in learning. *Early Years, 32(1)*: 17–34.

Garvey, C. (1991). *Play* (2nd edn). London: Fontana Press.

Gerhardt, S. (2004). *Why Love Matters: How Affection Shapes a Baby's Brain*. London: Routledge.

Gill, T. (2007). *No Fear: Growing up in a Risk Averse Society*. London: Calouste Gulbenkian Foundation.

Gitlin-Weiner, K., Sandgrund, A. & Schaefer, C. (2002) *Play Diagnosis and Assessment*. London: John Wiley.

Gleave, J. (2008). *Risk and Play: A Literature Review*. London: Playday.

Gleave, J. & Cole-Hamilton, I. (2012). *A World without Play: A Literature Review*. London: Play England.

Goddard-Blythe, S. (2004). *The Well Balanced Child: Movement and Early Learning*. Gloucestershire: Hawthorn Press.

Goldschmied, E. & Jackson, S. (1994). *People Under Three: Young Children in Daycare*. London: Routledge.

Goouch, K. (2010). Permission to play. In J. Moyles (Ed.), *The Excellence of Play* (3rd edn) (pp. 53–66). Maidenhead: Open University Press.

Gopnik, A., Meltzoff, A. & Kuhl, P. (1999). *How Babies Think*. London: Weidenfeld & Nicolson.

Greenberg, M. T. (2006). Promoting resilience in children and youth: Preventative interventions and their interface with neuroscience. *Annals, New York Academy of Sciences, 1094*: 139–150.

Greenspan, S. (2003). *Engaging Autism: The Floortime Approach to Helping Children Relate, Communicate and Think*. Jackson, TN: Perseus Books.

Guitard, P., Ferland, F. & Dutil, E. (2005). Towards a better understanding of playfulness in adults. *OTJR: Occupation, Participation and Health, 25(1)*: 9–22.

Hallam, S. (2010). The power of music: Its impact on the intellectual, social and personal development of children and young people. *International Journal of Music Education, 28(3)*: 269–289.

Hamm, E. M. (2006). Playfulness and the environmental support of play in children with and without developmental disabilities. *OTJR: Occupation, Participation and Health, 26(3)*: 88–96.

Hendry, L. B. & Kloep, M. (2002). *Lifespan Development: Resources, Challenge and Risk*. Andover: Cengage Learning EMEA.

Herbert, M. (2003). *Typical and Atypical Development*. London: Blackwell.

Hewett, D. & Nind, M. (2005). *Access to Communication: Developing Basic Communication with People who have Severe Learning Difficulties*. New York: David Fulton.

Hill, M., Head, G., Lockyer, A., Reid, B. & Taylor, R. (2012). *Children's Services: Working Together*. London: Pearson.

Holmes, R. M. (1999). Kindergarten and college students' views of play and work at home and at school. In S. Reifel (Ed.), *Play and Culture Studies* (Vol. 2, pp. 59–72). Stanford, CT: Ablex Publishing Corporation.

Howard, J. (2002). Eliciting young children's perceptions of play, work and learning using the activity apperception story procedure. *Early Child Development and Care, 172*: 489–502.

Howard, J. (2010a). Making the most of play in the early years. In P. Broadhead, J. Howard & E. Wood (Eds), *Play and Learning in the Early Years* (pp. 145–160). London: Sage Publishing Ltd.

Howard, J. (2010b). Early years practitioners' perceptions of play: An exploration of theoretical understanding, planning and involvement, confidence and barriers to practice. *Child and Educational Psychology, 27(4)*: 91–112.

Howard, J. (2010c). The development and therapeutic potential of play: Re-establishing teachers as play professionals. In J. Moyles (Ed.), *The Excellence of Play* (3rd edn) (pp. 201–215). Maidenhead: Open University Press.

Howard, J. & Elton, H. (2009). *Measuring Children's Heights and Weights in Wales: Report to the Welsh Assembly Government to Inform the Minister for Health and Social Services on the Findings from a Study to Explore the Feasibility of a National Measurement Programme and Recommendations for Future Rollout Across Wales: Consulting Children Element*. NPHS.

Howard, J. & McInnes, K. (2012). The impact of children's perceptions of an activity as play rather than not play on emotional well-being. *Child: Care, Health and Development*, 6 June. doi: 10.1111/j.1365-2214.2012.01405.x.

Howard, J. & Westcott, M. (2007). Research into practice: Creating a playful classroom environment. *Psychology of Education Review, 31(1)*: 27–34.

Howard, J., Jenvey, V. & Hill, C. (2006). Children's categorisation of play and learning based on social context. *Early Child Development and Care, 176(3&4)*: 379–393.

Howard, J., Miles, G. & Parker, C. (2008). Understanding children's perceptions of play using the Revised Apperception Procedure: Implications for practice in early years settings. Paper presented at EECERA, Norway, September.

Howard, J., Miles, G. & Rees-Davies, L. (2012). Computer use within a play-based early years curriculum. *International Journal of Early Years Education* (accepted, forthcoming 2012).

Howe, D. (2006). Developmental attachment psychotherapy with fostered and adopted children. *Child and Adolescent Mental Health, 11(3)*: 128–134.

Hughes, B. (2001). *Evolutionary Playwork and Reflective Analytic Practice*. London: Routledge.

Hughes, B. (2006). *Play Types: Speculations and Possibilities*. London: Centre for Playwork Education and Training.

Hughes, B. (2011). Playing into the future – surviving and thriving. Paper presented at the IPA World Conference.

Hughes, F. P. (2010). *Children, Play and Development* (4th edn). London: Sage Publications Ltd.

Humphrey, N., Kalambouka, A., Bolton, J., Lendrum, L., Wigelsworth, M., Lennie, C. & Farrell, P. (2010). *Social and Emotional Aspects of Learning (SEAL): Evaluation of Small Group Work*. Research Report, DCSF RR064.

Hutt, C. (1976). Exploration and play in children. In J. S. Bruner, A. Jolly & K. Sylva (Eds), *Play: Its Role in Development and Evolution* (pp. 202–215). Harmondsworth: Penguin Books Ltd.

Hutt, S. J., Tyler, S., Hutt, C. & Christopherson, H. (1989). *Play, Exploration and Learning*. London: Routledge.

Isaacs, S. (1929). *The Nursery Years*. London: Routledge & Kegan Paul.

Isaacs, S. (1932). *The Children We Teach*. London: University of London Press Ltd.

James, A., Jenks, C. & Prout, A. (1998). *Theorising Childhood*. Oxford: Polity Press.

James, W. (1981). *The Principles of Psychology*. Cambridge, MA: Harvard University Press [first published in 1890].

Jarrold, C. (2003). A review of research into pretend play in autism. *Autism, 7*: 379–390.

Jarvis, P. (2006). Rough and tumble play: Lessons in life. *Evolutionary Psychology, 4*: 330–346.

Jarvis, P. (2009). Play, narrative and learning in education: A biocultural perspective. *Education & Child Psychology, 26(2)*: 66–76.

Jennings, S. (1999). *Introduction to Developmental Playtherapy*. London: Jessica Kingsley Press.

Johnson, J. E., Christie, J. F. & Wardle, F. (2005). *Play, Development and Early Education*. Boston, MA: Pearson Education, Inc.

Jones, E. & Reynolds, G. (1992). *The Play's the Thing . . . Teachers' Roles in Children's Play*. New York: Teachers College Press.

Karrby, G. (1989). Children's conceptions of their own play. *International Journal of Early Childhood Education, 21(2)*: 49–54.

Katz, L. G. (1993). Dispositions as educational goals. *Journal*, 1–5. Retrieved from: www.eric.ed.gov.

Keating, I., Fabian, H., Jordan, P., Mavers, D. & Roberts, J. (2000). 'Well, I've not done any work today. I don't know why I came to school': Perceptions of play in the reception class. *Educational Studies, 26(4)*: 437–454.

Kelly-Vance, L. & Ryalls, B. (2008). Best practices in play assessment and intervention. In *Best Practices in School Psychology* (5th edn) (Volume 2, pp. 549–560). Bethesda, MD: National Association of School Psychologists.

King, N. R. (1979). Play: The kindergartners' perspective. *The Elementary School Journal, 80(2)*: 81–87.

King, P. & Howard, J. (2012). Children's perceptions of choice in relation to their play at home, in the school playground and at the out-of-school club. *Children & Society,* doi:10.1111/j.1099-0860.2012.00455.x.

Kirby, A. (2006). *Dyspraxia: Developmental Co-ordination Disorder*. London: Souvenir Press.

Kose, G., Beilin, H. & O'Connor, J. M. (1983). Children's comprehension of actions depicted in photographs. *Developmental Psychology, 19(4)*: 636–643.

Krasnor, L. R. & Pepler, D. J. (1980). The study of children's play: Some suggested future directions. In K. H. Rubin (Ed.), *New Directions for Child Development: Children's Play* (Vol. 9, pp. 85–95). San Francisco: Jossey-Bass Inc. Publishers.

Kytta, M. (2004). The extent of children's independent mobility and the number of actualised affordances as criteria for child-friendly environments. *Journal of Environmental Psychology, 24*: 179–198.

Laevers, F. (2008). The Project Experiential Education: Concepts and experiences at the level of context, process and outcome. Retrieved from http://european-agency.org/agency-projects/assessmentresource-guide/documents/2008/11/Laevers.pdf.

Laevers, F., Vandenbussche, E., Kog, M. & Depondt, L. (1994). *A Process-Oriented Child Monitoring System for Young Children*. Leuven, Belgium: Centre for Experiental Education.

Landreth, G. L. (2012). *Play Therapy: The Art of the Relationship* (3rd edn). New York: Routledge.

Layard, R. & Dunn, J. (2009). *A Good Childhood*. London: Penguin Books.

Lee, N. (2002). *Childhood and Society: Growing Up in an Age of Uncertainty*. Buckingham: Open University Press.

Lester, S. & Russell, W. (2008). *Play for a Change*. London: Play England/National Children's Bureau.

Lester, S. & Russell, W. (2010). Children's right to play: An examination of the importance of play in the lives of children worldwide. *Working Papers in Early Childhood Development (57)*. The Hague, Netherlands: Bernard Van Leer Foundation

Li, W. & Lopez, V. (2008). Effectiveness and appropriateness of therapeutic play intervention in preparing children for surgery: A randomized controlled trial study. *Journal for Specialists in Pediatric Nursing, 13(2)*: 63–73.

Lieberman, J. N. (1977). *Playfulness: Its Relationship to Imagination and Creativity*. New York: Academic Press Inc.

Lowenfeld, M. (1979). *The World Technique*. London: Allen & Unwin.

Luckett, T., Bundy, A. & Roberts, J. (2007). Do behavioural approaches teach children with autism to play or are they pretending? *Autism, 11*: 365–388.

Ludemos Associates (2008–11). Ludemos. Accessed from: http://www.ludemos.co.uk/Psycholudics%20-%20Terminology%206%202011.pdf [retrieved 2 August 2011].

MacBeath, J., Galton, M., Steward, S., MacBeath, A. & Page, C. (2006). *The Costs of Inclusion: A Study of Inclusion Policy and Practice in English Primary, Secondary and Special Schools*. Cambridge: Victoire Press.

Manning, K. C, & Sharp, A. (1977). *Structuring Play in the Early Years at School*. East Grinstead: Schools Council Publications.

Manwaring, B. (2006). *Children's Views 2006: Children and Young People's Views on Play and Playworkers*. http://playbristol.org/static/uploads/1257947368-child.pdf.

Masten A. (2001). Ordinary magic: Resilience processes in development. *American Psychologist, 56(3)*: 227–238.

Masten, A. & Coatsworth, J. (1998). The development of competence in favorable and unfavorable environments. *American Psychologist, 53(2)*: 205–220.

McInnes, K., Howard, J., Miles, G. E. & Crowley, K. (2009). Behavioural differences exhibited by children when practising a task under formal and playful conditions. *Educational & Child Psychology, 26(2)*: 31–39.

McInnes, K., Howard, J., Miles, G. E. & Crowley, K. (2010). Differences in adult–child interactions during playful and formal practice conditions: An initial investigation. *The Psychology of Education Review, 34(1)*: 14–20.

McInnes, K., Howard, J., Miles, G. E. & Crowley, K. (2011). Differences in practitioners' understanding of play and how this influences pedagogy and children's perceptions of play. *Early Years: An International Journal of Research and Development, 31(2)*: 121–133.

McInnes, K., Howard, J., Crowley, K. & Miles, G. (in press). The nature of adult–child interaction in the early years classroom: Implications for children's perceptions of play and subsequent learning behaviour. *European Early Childhood Education Research Journal*.

McMahon, L. (2009). *The Handbook of Play Therapy and Therapeutic Play* (2nd edn). London: Routledge.

Meltzoff, A. N. & Moore, M. K. (1999). Persons and representation: Why infant imitation is important for theories of human development. In J. Nadel & G. Butterworth (Eds), *Imitation in Infancy*. Cambridge Studies in Cognitive Perceptual Development (pp. 9–35). New York: Cambridge University Press.

Montessori, M. (1965). *Dr. Montessori's Own Handbook*. New York: Shocken Books Inc.

Moyles, J. R. (1989). *Just Playing?* Buckingham: Open University Press.

Neumann, E. A. (1971). *The Elements of Play*. New York: MSS Information Corporation.

NICE (National Institute for Health and Clinical Excellence) (2008). Promoting children's social and emotional wellbeing in primary education. *Journal*. Retrieved from www.nice.org.uk/PH012.

Nicholson, S. (1971). The theory of loose parts. *Landscape Architecture Quarterly, 62(1)*: 30–34.

Niklasson, M., Niklasson, I. & Norlander, T. (2010). Sensorimotor therapy: Physical and psychological regressions contribute to an improved kinesthetic and vestibular capacity in children and adolescents with motor difficulties and concentration problems. *Social Behaviour and Personality 38(3)*: 327–345.

Nutbrown, C. & Clough, P. (2009). Citizenship and inclusion in the early years: Understanding and responding to children's perspectives on 'belonging'. *International Journal of Early Years Education, 17(3)*: 191–206.

Oaklander, V. (1988). *Windows to Our Children*. Highland, NY: The Gestalt Journal Press.

ODI (Office for Disability Issues) (2010). *The Life Opportunities of Disabled People: Qualitative Research on Choice and Control and Access to Goods and Services*. London: HMSO.

Orr, R. (2003). *My Right to Play: A Child with Complex Needs*. Buckingham: Open University Press.

Owen-Leeds, L. (2012). Understanding older children's perceptions of play and subsequently manipulating the cues: The effectiveness of playful practice for problem-solving. Unpublished BSc Dissertation, University of Glamorgan.

Palmer, S. (2006). *Toxic Childhood*. London: Orion.

Panksepp, J. (2007). Can play diminish ADHD and facilitate the development of the social brain? *Journal of the Canadian Academy of Child and Adolescent Psychiatry, 16(2)*: 57–66.

Parker, C. (2007). Children's perceptions of a playful environment: Contextual, social and environmental differences. Unpublished Bachelor's Thesis, University of Glamorgan.

Parker-Rees, R. (1999). Protecting playfulness. In L. Abbott & H. Moylett (Eds), *Early Education Transformed* (pp. 61–72). London: Falmer Press.

Parten, M. (1932). Social participation among preschool children. *Journal of Abnormal and Social Psychology, 28(3)*: 136–147.

Patel, A., Schieble, T., Davidson, M., Tran, M., Schoenberg, C., Delphin, E. & Bennett, H. (2006). Distraction with a hand-held video game reduces pediatric preoperative anxiety. *Paediatric Anaesthesia, 16(10)*: 1019–1027.

Pellegrini, A. D. (1991). *Applied Child Study* (2nd edn). Hillsdale, NJ: Lawrence Erlbaum Associates, Inc.

Pellegrini, A. D. (2009). *The Role of Play in Human Development*. Oxford: Oxford University Press.

Piaget, J. (1951). *Play, Dreams and Imitation in Childhood*. London: William Heinemann Ltd.

Play England (2010). *Making the Case for Play*. Available from: http://www.playengland. org.uk/media/261359/scp-action-pack-making-the-case.pdf [retrieved 20 April 2012].

Porter, J., Daniels, H., Georgeson, J., Hacker, J., Gallo, V., Feiler, A., Tarleto, B. & Watson, D. (2008). *Disability Data Collection for Children's Services*. DCSF Research Report RR062, Nottingham.

Powell, S. & Wellard, I. (2008). *Policies and Play: The Impact of National Policies on Opportunities for Children's Play*. London: National Children's Bureau.

Ring, K. (2010). Keeping it playful: Adults supporting young children making meaning through drawing in Foundation Stage contexts. In P. Broadhead, J. Howard & E. Woods (Eds), *Play and Learning in the Early Years*. London: Sage Publications.

Robson, S. (1993). 'Best of all I like choosing time': Talking with children about play and work. *Early Child Development and Care, 92*: 37–51.

Robson, S. (2011). Using video data with young children. In D. Harcourt, B. Perry & T. Waller (Eds), *Researching Young Children's Perspectives* (pp. 178–192). London: Routledge.

Roeyers, H. & Van Berkalaer-Onnes, I. (1994). Play in autistic children. *Communication and Cognition, 27*: 349–359.

Rogers, C. (1951). *Client-Centered Therapy: Its Current Practice, Implications and Theory*. London: Constable.

Rogers, C. S. & Sluss, D. J. (1999). Play and inventiveness: Revisiting Erikson's views on Einstein's playfulness. In S. Reifel (Ed.), *Play and Culture Studies. Volume 2* (Vol. 2, pp. 3–24). Stamford, CT: Ablex Publishing Corporation.

Rogoff, B. (2003). *The Cultural Nature of Human Development*. New York: Oxford University Press.

Rothlein, L. & Brett, A. (1987). Children's, teachers' and parents' perceptions of play. *Early Childhood Research Quarterly, 2*: 45–53.

Rubin, K. H., Fein, G. G. & Vandenberg, B. (1983). Play. In P. H. Mussen (Ed.), *Handbook of Child Psychology, 4th Edition. Vol. IV: Socialisation, Personality and Social Development* (pp. 694–759). New York: John Wiley & Sons.

Rutter, M., Kim-Cohen, J. & Maughan, B. (2006). Continuities and discontinuities in psychopathology between childhood and adult life. *Journal of Child Psychology and Psychiatry, 47(3)*: 276–295.

Sameroff, A. (2010). A unified theory of development: A dialectic integration of nature and nurture. *Child Development, 81(1)*: 6–22.

Sandseter, E. (2007). Categorising risky play: How can we identify risk taking in children's play? *European Early Childhood Research, 15(2)*: 237–252.

Saracho, O. N. & Spodek, B. (1998). A historical overview of theories of play. In O. N. Saracho & B. Spodek (Eds), *Multiple Perspectives on Play in Early Childhood Education* (pp. 1–10). Albany, NY: State University of New York Press.

Schaefer, C. (2011). *Foundations of Play Therapy*. New York: John Wiley.

Schaefer, C. & Greenberg, R. (1997). Measurement of playfulness: A neglected therapist variable. *International Journal of Play Therapy, 6(2)*: 21–31.

Schirrmacher, R. (2002). *Art and Creative Development for Young Children* (4th edn). Albany, NY: Delmar Thomson Learning.

Shaaf, R. & Miller, L. (2005). Occupational Therapy using a sensory integration approach for children with developmental disabilities. *Mental Retardation and Developmental Disabilities Research Reviews, 11*: 143–148.

Sheridan, M., Howard, J. & Alderson, D. (2010). *Play in Early Childhood* (3rd edn). London: Routledge.

Singer, J. S. & Singer, D. G. (1980). A factor analytic study of preschoolers' play behaviour. *Academic Psychology Bulletin, 2* (June): 143–156.

Skeate, F. (2011). Exploring the effects of an intensive play training programme for practitioners caring for children in residential care homes. Unpublished Master's Thesis, Swansea University.

Skybo, T., Wenger, N. & Su, Y. (2007). Human figure drawings as a measure of children's emotional status: Critical review for practice. *Journal of Pediatric Nursing, 22(1)*: 15–28.

Smidt, S. (2011). *Playing to Learn: The Role of Play in the Early Years*. London: Routledge.

Smilansky, S. (1968). *The Effects of Sociodramatic Play on Disadvantaged Preschool Children*. New York: John Wiley & Sons Ltd.

Smith, P. K. (2010). *Children and Play*. Chichester: Wiley-Blackwell.

Smith, P. K. & Whitney, S. (1987). Play and associative fluency: Experimenter effects may be responsible for previous positive findings. *Developmental Psychology, 23(1)*: 49–53.

Smith, P. K., Takhvar, M., Gore, N. & Vollstedt, R. (1986). Play in young children: Problems of definition, categorisation and measurement. In P. K. Smith (Ed.), *Children's Play: Research Developments and Practical Applications* (pp. 39–55). London: Gordon & Breach Science Publishers.

Special Needs and Disability Act (2001) [online] HMSO2001 (c.10). Available from: www.hmso.gov.uk.

Stagnitti, K. & Cooper, R. (2009). *Play as Therapy: Assessment and Therapeutic Interventions*. London: Jessica Kingsley Press.

Stallibrass, A. (1977). *The Self-Respecting Child*. Harmondsworth: Penguin Books Ltd.

Stephenson, A. (2003). Physical risk-taking: dangerous or endangered? *Early Years, 23(1)*: 35–43.

Sturgess, J. & Ziviani, J. (1996). A self-report play skills questionnaire: Technical development. *Australian Occupational Therapy Journal, 43*: 142–154.

Sturrock, G. & Else, P. (1998). The playground as therapeutic space: Playwork as healing [known as the 'Colorado Paper']. In G. Sturrock and P. Else (2005) *Therapeutic Playwork: Reader One*. Sheffield: Ludemos.

Sunderland, M. (2001). *Using Storytelling as a Therapeutic Tool with Children*. Milton Keynes: Speechmark Publishing.

Sutton-Smith, B. (Ed.) (1979). *Play and Learning*. New York: Gardnet Press Inc.

Sutton-Smith, B. (1997). *The Ambiguity of Play*. Cambridge, MA: Harvard University Press.

Sutton-Smith, B. (2003). Play as a parody of emotional vulnerability. In J. Roopnarine (Ed.), *Play and Educational Theory and Practice*. Play and Culture Studies, Vol. 5. Westport, CT: Praeger

Sutton-Smith, B. & Kelly-Byrne, D. (1984). The idealization of play. In P. K. Smith (Ed.), *Play in Animals and Humans* (pp. 305–321). Oxford: Basil Blackwell Ltd.

Tegano, D. W. (1990). Relationship of tolerance of ambiguity and playfulness to creativity. *Psychological Reports, 66*: 1047–1056.

Thomas, L., Howard, J. & Miles, G. (2006). The effectiveness of playful practice for learning in the early years. *The Psychology of Education Review, 30(1)*: 52–58.

Thompson, J., Coon, K., Boddy, K., Stein, R., Whear, J., Barton, M. & Depledge, H. (2011). Does participating in physical activity in outdoor natural environments have a greater effect on physical and mental wellbeing than physical activity indoors? A systematic review. *Environmental Science and Technology, 45(5)*: 1761–1772.

Timberlake, E. M. & Cutler, M. M. (2001). *Developmental Play Therapy in Clinical Social Work*. Needham Heights, MA: Allyn & Bacon.

Tovey, H. (2007). *Playing Outdoor: Spaces and Places, Risk and Challenge*. Maidenhead: Open University Press.

Tovey, H. (2010). Playing on the edge: Perceptions of risk and danger in outdoor play. In P. Broadhead, J. Howard & E. Wood (Eds), *Play and Learning in the Early Years*. London: Sage Publications Ltd.

UNICEF (2009). United Nations Convention on the Rights of the Child. www.unicef.org.uk/tz/rights.convention.asp [accessed 9 June 2010].

Valentine, G. (2004). *Public Spaces and the Culture of Childhood*. Aldershot: Ashgate.

Valsiner, J. (2000). *Culture and Human Development*. London: Sage.

Van Fleet, R. (2005). *Filial Therapy: Strengthening Parent–Child Relationships Through Play* (2nd edn). Sarasota, FL: Professional Resource Press.

VanHoorn, K., Nourot, P. M., Scales, P. M. & Alward, K. R. (2007). *Play at the Center of the Curriculum*. Upper Saddle River, NJ: Pearson.

Vygotsky, L. S. (1933). Play and its role in the mental development of the child. *Journal*. Retrieved from: http://www.marxists.org/archive/vygotsky/works/1933/play.htm.

Vygotsky, L. S. (1978). *Mind and Society: The Development of Higher Psychological Processes*. Cambridge, MA: Harvard University Press.

Walsh, G., Sproule, L., McGuinesss, C. & Trew, K. (2011). Playful structure: A novel image of early years pedagogy for primary school classrooms. *Early Years, 31 (2)*: 107–119.

Waters, J. & Begley, S. (2007). Supporting the development of risk-taking behaviour in the early years: An exploratory study. *Education 3–13, 35(4)*: 365–377.

Watson, J. B. & Rayner, R. (1920). Conditioned emotional reactions. *Journal of Experimental Psychology, 3(1)*: 1–14.

Welsh Assembly Government (2011). *Child Poverty Strategy for Wales*. Available from: www.wales.gov.uk/educationandskills.

Welsh Assembly Government (2012). *Play: Health and Wellbeing*. Available from: www.playwales.org.uk.

West, J. (1996). *Child Centred Play Therapy* (2nd edn). London: Hodder Arnold.

West-Burnham, J. (2008). *Leadership for Personalised Learning*. Nottingham: NCSL.

Westcott, H. L. & Littleton, K. S. (2005). Exploring meaning in interviews with children. In S. Greene & D. Hogan (Eds), *Researching Children's Experience: Approaches and Methods* (pp. 141–157). London: Sage Publications Ltd.

White, D. (2012). Differences in primary school teachers' and playworkers' views on children's play and how this influences their practice. Unpublished BSc Dissertation, University of Glamorgan.

Whitebread, D. (2012). *Developmental Psychology & Early Childhood Education*. London: Sage Publications Ltd.

Whitebread, D., Basilio, M., Kuvalja, M. & Verma, M. (2012). *The Value of Children's Play*. A report written for the Toy Industries of Europe. University of Cambridge.

Williams, J. & McInnes, K. (2005). *Planning and Using Time in the Foundation Stage*. London: David Fulton Publishers.

Wing, L. (1995). Play is not the work of the child: Young children's perceptions of work and play. *Early Childhood Research Quarterly, 10*: 223–247.

Wing, L. & Gould, J. (1979). Severe impairments of social interaction and associated abnormalities in children: Epidemiology and classification. *Journal of Autism and Developmental Disorders, 9*: 11–30.

Winnicott, D. W. (1971). *Playing and Reality*. London: Routledge Classics.

Wood, E. (2010). Reconceptualizing the play–pedagogy relationship: From control to complexity. In E. Brooker & S. Edwards (Eds), *Engaging Play*. Maidenhead: McGraw-Hill.

Wood, E. & Attfield, J. (2005). *Play, Learning and the Early Childhood Curriculum* (2nd edn). London: Paul Chapman Publishing.

Worthington, M. (2007). Multi-modality, play and children's mark-making in maths. In J. Moyles (Ed.), *Early Years Foundations: Meeting the Challenge*. Maidenhead: Open University Press.

Yarnal, C. & Qian, X. (2011). Older-adult playfulness: An innovative construct and measurement for healthy aging research. *American Journal of Play, 4(1)*: 52–79.

Youell, B. (2009). The importance of play and playfulness. In R. House and D.

Lowenthal (Eds), *Childhood, Wellbeing and Therapeutic Ethos*. London: Karnac Books.

Young, T., Griffin, E., Phillips, E. & Stanley, E. (2010). Music as a distraction in a paediatric emergency department. *Journal of Emergency Nursing, 36(5)*: 472–473.

Zeanah, C.H., Smyke, A., Koga, S. & Carlson, E. (2005). Attachment in institutionalised and community children in Romania. *Child Development, 76(5)*: 1015–1028.

Zosuls, K. (2009). The acquisition of gender labels in infancy: Implications for sex typed play. *Developmental Psychology, 45(3)*: 688–701.

Index